WEIGHT LOSS

WITH

MENTAL DIEt

THE COMPLETE GUIDE TO LOSE WEIGHT STEP BY STEP THROUGH THE POWER OF MIND

Melanie Johnson

Melanie Johnson

Melanie Johnson

Table of Contents

Melanie Johnson

Introduction

There are many contradictions in the history of hypnosis. Its history is a bit like trying to find the history of breathing. Hypnosis is a universal trait that was built in at birth. It has been experienced and shared by every human since the beginning of time. It has just been in the past few decades that we are beginning to understand this. Hypnosis hasn't changed in a million years. The way we understand it and how we control it has changed a lot.

Hypnosis has always been surrounded by misconceptions and myths. Despite being used clinically and all the research that has been done, some continue to be scared by the assumption that hypnosis is mystical. Many people think that hypnosis is a modern-day innovation that spread through communities that believed in the metaphysical during the 70s and 80s. Since the mid-1800s, hypnosis was used in the United States. It has advanced with the help of psychologists such as Alfred Binet, Pierre Janet, and Sigmund Freud, and others. Hypnosis can be found in ancient times and has been investigated by modern researchers, physicians, and psychologists.

Hypnosis's origins can't be separated from psychology and western medicine. Most ancient cultures from Roman, Greek, Egyptian, Indian, Chinese, Persian, and Sumerian used hypnosis. In Greece and Egypt, people who were sick would go to the places that healed. These were known as dream temples or sleep temples where people could be cured with hypnosis. The Sanskrit book called "The Law of Manu" described levels of hypnosis such as sleep-walking, dream sleep, and ecstasy sleep in ancient India.

The earliest evidence of hypnosis was found in the Egyptian Ebers Papyrus that dated back to 1550 BC. Priest/physicians repeated suggestions while treating patients. They would have the patient gaze at metal discs and enter a trance. This is now called eye fixation.

During the Middle Ages, princes and kings thought they could heal with the Royal Touch. These healings can be attributed to divine powers. Before people began to understand hypnosis, the terms mesmerism or magnetism would be used to describe this type of healing.

Melanie Johnson

Paracelsus, the Swiss physician, began using magnets to heal. He didn't use a holy relic or divine touch. This type of healing was still being used in the 1700s. A Jesuit priest, Maximillian Hell, was famous for healing using magnetic steel plates. Franz Mesmer, an Austrian physician, discovered he could send people into a trance without the use of magnets. He found out the healing force came from inside himself or an invisible fluid that took up space. He thought that "animal magnetism" could be transferred from the patient to healer by a mysterious etheric fluid. This theory is so wrong. It was based on ideas that were current during the time, specifically Isaac Newton's theory of gravity.

Mesmer developed a method for hypnosis that was passed on to his followers. Mesmer would perform inductions by linking his patients together by a rope that the animal magnetism could pass over. He would also wear a cloak and play music on a glass harmonica while all this was happening.

These practices led to his downfall, and for time hypnotism was considered dangerous for anyone to have as a career. The fact remains that hypnosis works. The 19th century was full of people who were looking to understand and apply it.

Marquis de Puysegur, a student of Mesmer, was a successful magnetist who first used hypnosis called somnambulism or sleepwalking. Puysegur's followers called themselves experimentalists. Their work recognized that cures didn't come from magnets but an invisible source.

Abbe Faria, an Indo-Portuguese priest, did hypnosis research in India during 1813. He went to Paris and studied hypnosis with Puysegur. He thought that hypnosis or magnetism wasn't what healed but the power that was generated from inside the mind.

His approach was what helped open the psychotherapy hypnosis centered school called Nancy School. The Nancy School said that hypnosis was a phenomenon brought on by the power of suggestion and not from magnetism. This school was founded by a French country doctor, Ambroise-Auguste Liebeault. He was called the father of modern hypnotherapy. He thought hypnosis was psychological and had nothing to do with magnetism. He studied the similar qualities of trance and sleep and noticed that hypnosis was a state that could be brought on my suggestion.

His book Sleep and Its Analogous States, was printed in 1866. The stories and writings about his cures attracted

Hippolyte Bernheim to visit him. Bernheim was a famous neurologist who was skeptical of Liebeault, but once he observed Liebault, he was so intrigued that he gave up internal medicine and became a hypnotherapist. Bernheim brought Liebeault's ideas to the medical world with Suggestive Therapeutics that showed hypnosis as a science. Bernheim and Liebeault were the innovators of psychotherapy. Even today, hypnosis is still viewed as a phenomenon.

The pioneers of psychology studied hypnosis in Paris and Nancy Schools. Pierre Janey developed theories of traumatic memory, dissociation, and unconscious processes studied hypnosis with Bernheim in Charcot in Paris and Nancy. Sigmund Freud studied hypnosis with Charcot and observed both Liebeault and Bernheim.

Melanie Johnson

Freud started practicing hypnosis in 1887. Hypnosis was critical in him invented psychoanalysis.

During the time that hypnosis was being invented, several physicians began using hypnosis for anesthesia. Recamier, in 1821 operated while using hypnosis as anesthesia. John Elliotson, a British surgeon in 1834, introduced the stethoscope in England. He reported doing several painless operations by using hypnosis. A Scottish surgeon, James Esdaile, did over 345 major and 2,000 minor operations by using hypnosis during the 1840s and 1850s.

James Braid, a Scottish ophthalmologist, invented modern hypnotism. Braid first used the term nervous sleep or neuro-hypnotism that became hypnosis or hypnotism. Braid went to a demonstration of La Fontaine, the French magnetism in 1841. He ridiculed the Mesmerists' ideas and suggested that hypnosis was psychological. He was the first to practice psychosomatic medicine. He tried to say that hypnosis was just focusing on one idea. Hypnosis was advanced by the Nancy School and is still a term we use today.

The center of hypnosis moved out of Europe and into America. Here it had many breakthroughs in the 20th century. Hypnosis was a popular phenomenon that because more available to normal people who were not doctors. Hypnosis's style changed, too. It was no longer direct instructions from an authority; instead, it became more of a permissive and indirect style of trance that was based on subtle language patterns. This was brought about by Milton H. Erickson. Using hypnosis for quick treatment of trauma and injuries during WWI,

WWII, and Korea led to a new interest in hypnosis in psychiatry and dentistry.

Hypnosis started becoming more practical and was thought of as a tool for helping psychological distress. Advances in brain imaging and neurological science, along with Ivan Tyrrell and Joe Griffin's work, have helped resolve some debates. These British psychologists linked hypnosis to Rapid Eye Movement and brought hypnosis into the realm of daily experiences. The nature of normal consciousness can be understood better as just trance states that we constantly go in and out of.

There are still people who think that hypnosis is a type of power held by the occult even today. The people that believe hypnosis can control minds or perform miracles are sharing the views that have been around for hundreds of years. The history that has been recorded is rich with glimpses of practices and ancient rituals that look like modern hypnosis. The Hindu Vedas have healing passes. Ancient Egypt has its magical texts. These practices were used for religious ceremonies, like communicating with spirits and gods. We need to remember that what people view as the occult was science at its finest in that time frame. It was doing the same thing as modern science was doing now trying to cure human ailments by increasing our knowledge.

Finding the history of hypnosis is like searching for something that is right in our view. We can begin to see it for what it actually is – a phenomenon that is a complicated part of human existence. Hypnosis's future is to completely realize our natural hypnotic abilities and the potential we all hold inside us.

Melanie Johnson

For so many years now, individuals have been contemplating and contending about this topic. All hypnosis scientists are yet to explain how it really works. With hypnosis, you'll be able to see an individual under a trance, but you won't understand what is going on. This trance is a little piece of how human personality works. It is safe to say that hypnosis will continue to remain a mystery to us. We all know the general aspects of hypnosis, but we can't truly understand how it works. Hypnosis is a condition of series portrayed by serious suggestive expanded and unwinding dreams. It is not sleeping, because when you are under hypnosis, you are still under alert. But you are simply wondering into fantasyland, and you feel yourself going into another dimension that is different from this physical dimension.

Melanie Johnson

You are completely mindful, but you are not mindful of the environment around you. You are only mindful of that thing that is being portrayed in your mind and that dreamland that you are going into. In your normal day of life, you can feel the universe and the universe effect on your feelings. Research has shown that hypnosis can be used to cure several conditions. It is effective in elevating conditions like rheumatism joint pains. It helps to elevate labor pains and childbearing pains. It has also been used to reduce diamante side effects. It also helps in ADHD side effects hypnotherapy. And it reduces the impact of sickness in the body. It also helps during torment. It can also help to improve dental pains and skin conditions like moles.

It also helps to cure disorder manifestation. Also, it can be used to ease the torment of agony brought about by childbirth and childbearing. It also helps to cure smoking, reduce weight, and stop bedwetting.

Melanie Johnson

Chapter 1: Instructions to Make the Most of Hypnosis and Lose Weight

They say we only use about 10% of our brains. That may be real, but I'd rather look at it differently. Consider 10 percent of your conscious mind. In other words, that part generates what you want, the part that thinks about you, analyzes what's going on, makes decisions and is your will power. So, it's a powerful mind pair.

But where's the mind's other 90%? Imagine the subconscious part. It's different from the conscious component. It doesn't think so. This holds all of your ideals, convictions, behaviors, history, and much more. That's the mental part that really regulates you.

Once you've learned to ride a bike and balanced, you'll never forget. If you haven't been on for a while, you may be out of practice, but once you get on your subconscious, you get into gear, and you're able to balance and ride really quickly.

The subconscious is computer-like. When you've programmed it, you'll get what you put in it. When your subconscious mind is full of trash and things you don't like, then that's what it's going to give you. It doesn't think eating when you're full is evil. It's just because, in the past, you designed it that way.

If the subconscious is about 90% of the mind and therefore stronger, why does it not respond to what the imaginative analytical conscious mind says? It's all about what you know and says it. Imagine a 7-year-old. She can be really supportive, or she can dig her heels down, not do what you want, and ignore you. When she's supportive, your mind's open to new ideas and improvement. Yet when she's unhelpful, avoiding the negative situation, that's different. When you try to tell her what you want, she'll probably forget you. When you try to push her to listen, it won't work either.

And how can you make changes to the subconscious? I use self-hypnosis myself, but if you haven't mastered it yet, you can use an affirmation instead. An affirmation is a constructive message you like. When you repeat an affirmation several times out loud, and to yourself, then the subconscious can note and take in what you affirm.

To make the affirmation function better and improve your mind's strength, you should do two things:

- Make sure the affirmation has some value for you. When you have eating disorders, and you make an affirmation, "I'm in control of my weight," the subconscious will forget the affirmation because it's not real. However, if you said, "I get more control of my eating habits every day," then work is more likely.

- Put as an issue. If you are seeking confirmation, the mind must first take it and find out what it means before it's real. It already starts after the affirmation and is real for you.

Conscious Mind and Subconscious Mind

Conscious Mind

The conscious mind can be compared to a word processor. It is the decision-maker for our day to day chores. This "processor" sends programs to the subconscious mind to perform certain tasks, observes how subconscious programs perform them, and then decides what else needs to be done.

The conscious mind is estimated to be only 12% of our minds. What it perceives as a belief is not exactly what our subconscious believes. You may think that there is absolutely no limitation in the subconscious for an issue, but they may still be there.

A unique quality of the conscious mind is that it can quickly judge what is right and what is wrong, something that the subconscious does not do. The conscious decide which information should be kept in the brain and which should not.

Subconscious Mind

Melanie Johnson

The subconscious mind is like a computer's hard drive. It contains memories, habits, beliefs, self-image and controls autonomous bodily functions. It is both the deposit of information and the executors of the tasks. It also contains "pre-defined instructions" that we don't have to consciously think about, such as keeping our heart beating, our breathing, our digestion...

The subconscious is estimated to be 88% of the mind. This means that when we recognize that one of our beliefs is negative, 12% of our mind wants to change the other 88%. Any decision to change is formed mainly in our conscious mind. This decision will, in some way, conflict with existing beliefs.

The subconscious mind's strength is incredible. By knowing the power of the inner mind, people can alter their unhappy life aspects. The subconscious mind occupies nearly all minds by about 88 percent. If people learn how to manage this subconscious mind properly, they can do everything in life. Your subconscious mind component represents personal patterns, temperament, and memory. And if you're looking for a positive shift of attitudes, actions or memory, then you have to focus on the subconscious mind.

The mind is closely associated with our experience, and it can show in the form of mental or physical disorder if we feed negative thoughts. Not letting negative thoughts spread in the subconscious mind. The future relies on people's thoughts and beliefs. If a person wants to win, they must have a winning attitude. Only then will they accomplish other things in life. It also gives positive inputs for positive output. Ignore negative thoughts because your subconscious mind cannot distinguish the difference between good or bad. So, thrive with good thoughts to increase the mind's healing power. Meditation and relaxation can effectively regulate the body.

Individuals can connect quickly with their subconscious mind using powerful affirmations. Affirmation is just constant reinforcement of optimistic thoughts. And it's really important to direct the good aspects. Through adding the strength of affirmations, people will strengthen their subconscious influence and boost enormous quantities of ability they never knew they had. And whatever the mind thinks it can do. Therefore, hitting the part of the subconscious mind may be a better way to expose the latent ability of the mind. So if people keep saying good thoughts constantly and holding faith in subconscious forces, they easily resolve their pain and hard times and pull circumstances that will make this conviction come true.

Subconscious mind strength is always misunderstood because people do not recognize their virtues. The part of the subconscious mind is the storage bank of all reinforcement (good or bad) we obtain in our surroundings. In adolescence, this affirmation directly affects one's behaviors. These same patterns decide our personality. To enhance our mind's capacity, feeding the right affirmation (repeatedly) into the subconscious is very necessary. This is possible with subliminal contact. People may write a tailor-made text message denoting positive affirmation. The encouragement is directed at the subconscious mind to develop a new habit. With age, developing new habits is extremely difficult for an aged person. Subliminal messaging can frame new habits. All of these allow for versatility to adapt to new behaviors. If properly used, the subconscious mind has forces far beyond human understanding. Uncover subconscious mind control by subliminal messaging.

Melanie Johnson

Melanie Johnson

Chapter 2: Ways to Use the Power of Your Mind to Increase Your Well-Being

We all want to feel good, love, have good jobs, etc. Those aspects are what most people around the world call "the good life." Though we all realize that being loved will not always make us feel good. This essay will explore the relationship between how we use our minds' strength and sense of well-being.

Well-being is not about physical comfort, but rather the far more profound concept of living a life that has a purpose, fulfilling your potential, or knowing how you make a positive difference in the world. People working in health care have a good attitude towards life in describing well-being as proof that we care for ourselves.

The "power of the mind" requires more than mental energy. Rather, it is a holistic concept that includes:

1) our being conscious and linked to the life force,

2) tracking minute emotional reactions to what is occurring at the moment, with the ability to

3) see, guide, and often direct our actions in the direction we believe would lead us to a more fulfilling existence.

It may be more appropriate to suggest that the power of our minds is our intellectual capacity to interpret and bring awareness to our existence as linked to the world around us — meaning that we are steering the ship, but it is also linked to the wider network of existence.

Melanie Johnson

Chapter 3: Why Can't You Lose Weight?

If you're like most people, you've lost weight just a few months down the road to gain it back. It is stressful and a growing problem. There are three main challenges I see people making while trying to lose weight to help you do better here: being too rigid with your plans. It's common knowledge that a person needs to minimize calories and exercise regularly to lose weight. Often people get fired up and fall into a rigid diet and exercise routine that isn't easy for life to manage. At first, it could be motivating, because you see some progress. The soreness in your muscles is beginning to fade, and you are feeling better. But it's challenging to carry on walking for an hour a day and watching what you eat, so you don't go over your daytime calories. We want to lose some pounds quickly, but the secret to keeping them off is to develop a balanced lifestyle that encourages you to enjoy eating and exercising. You're more likely to achieve your ideal healthier lifestyle. Applying carefulness strategies to your life can be a massive help in executing your plan without all the shame and judgement that often follows an overly rigorous diet and exercise program. The word "comfort food" is familiar to us. How do they reassure? Eating certain particular foods has a specific emotional connection, and they have little to do with hunger. Our minds establish relationships with things, objects, places and food that for different reasons are tucked away as good memories. The subconscious mind retains such convictions since they provide security in some way. Such beliefs are not always explicit, nor always make much sense at the moment. When we find those connections, we can use hypnosis research to rewire them to build new relationships which makes it easier to make healthier food choices, remove or minimize cravings and curb overeating.

Do not have a significant "Why"

Most people will lose a couple of pounds to get ready for a wedding, class reunion or holidays.

So far, we have seen some of the participants on The Biggest Loser that lost weight, looked terrific and enjoyed success after the contest ended only to revert to their old habits. Why? For what? It could be like they were in it because of the money and not because of the positive changes in life. Permanent weight loss is driven by a significant incentive to make the change. It could be a severe health problem that is the inspiration, maybe watching kids or grandchildren grow up or being able to engage more in life—seeking the "Why" for weight loss is an essential aspect of success. It is where coaching begins. You should work with a professional Life Coach to decide what's important to you, and that's what's most important to success. It's got to be necessary. You must decide you're going to eat healthily and you're going to exercise regularly, and you want to make those good habits a part of your life.

Once a person discovers a successful plan he/she can adapt, he/she acknowledges the emotional links to his/her eating patterns so that he/she can alter those feelings and relate it all to one or more significant reasons for making the positive adjustments that they are well on their road to success.

Why is weight regain underestimated?

Deprivation of calories leads to changes in metabolism, neutrality, and focus, and those changes make it challenging to indulge in the activities required to hold the weight off. Yet because such changes do not explicitly create pressure to return, a minority of dieters will still hold the weight off. That idea causes people to dismiss the current position of these improvements, and then argue that it must be due to their weak self-control if people get back weight. And since the modifications work by eating behavior, the weight loss does tend to be the result of the dieter's weak will. As many people have told me about unsuccessful dietitians, "they are always holding the fork." Here, the critical misconception is the specific physical and cognitive background in which dietitians keep the fork in contrast with non-dietitians: they feel hungry, their attention to food is skewed, they consider food tastier, and they get more pleasure from it. They tend to consume an even lower amount of food than they used to eat in the diet (as well as less than a non-dieter of the same size), as their more effective metabolism consumes fewer calories. So dieters don't have less willpower than non-dieters, but lack of calories has placed them in a position that takes much more willpower to reduce intake effectively.

Discover Over-Eating Causes.

The most effective method of weight reduction may be to find out what's making you overeat. A hypnotherapist will help you through the process and allow you the insight to problems and concerns you do not already know about.

Your hypnotherapist will be working as a mentor to help you through this process. The therapist should use carefully formulated instructions to find out what's bothering you by exploring hidden memories and your latent fears. Understanding the underlying causes of problems will allow you to once and for all old kick habits.

Melanie Johnson

Hypnotherapy will give you the support you need to get into shape and lose weight. Knowing what to expect and understanding how hypnotherapy can affect will provide you with the peace of mind, you need to go into a hypnosis session with confidence.

Have you attempted weight loss without success? Have you ever got the time to consider the preconscious and the emotional factors that could make you put on the weight?

Strong motivation and self-consciousness are both critical for positive results in reducing weight. Moreover, people who excel in weight-loss are potent believers in change. You might start attempting weight loss hypnosis to get in the right mindset.

Who Would Try Hypnosis?

Hypnosis is for those trying a gentle way to lose weight and make a habit of eating healthfully. For one guy, isn't it? Anyone wants a fast fix. This takes time to reframe negative feelings about food.

People's excuses struggle to lose weight.

1. Missed inspiration: Notwithstanding, seemingly every woman you meet complaining about her size and the shape – in fact most people are not serious about weight loss. The idea is that it is difficult to lose weight, will entail 'missing out' on foods you enjoy and will inevitably mean depriving yourself. This need not be the case with Hypnosis, the choice of how you change your behavior is entirely up to you as you are entirely in

control of your actions through the power of your unconscious mind.

2. Unrealistic Goals: Most of us just like the models and celebrities we see on TV and in magazines want to be the ideal size and form. Many people spend enormous amounts of energy, effort and resources in most situations – and could be blessed with significant genes too. We all want to look beautiful, slim and sexy, yeah, and please by the end of next week! And yet we are all of these things already – it is just that we forget sometimes. Weight loss is also about wanting to look healthy. Sometimes it is about feeling healthy. Hypnosis will also help you to understand your beauty and self-worth, and then build healthier behaviors to help you accomplish those things both within and outside!

3. Too early to give up: We just want to be slim-now! As soon as a, b, or c diet doesn't work for us within two flat days, we give up. "For me, it didn't fit". And yet it has taken us several months, even years to build up the excess weight. Hypnosis takes place immediately. The moment you listen is the moment you start to change your mind and therefore alter your behavior, and then the outcome will inevitably change. And all right, maybe by the end of the week, you won't be 14lbs lighter – but I've seen tests from a 7lbs client in a week before now! Yeah, and she said it was the best thing she ever could have done! This is workable stuff.

4. Not Healthy Eating: Most people can never get slim on chocolate, alcohol and fries because they're loaded with 'empty' calories that don't offer any nutritional value. The positive thing about these conventional diets

is they allow you to eat healthy – lots of fruits, vegetables and foods that are naturally low in fats. Hypnosis will help you make the right decisions for your loss of body, mind and weight – and yet let you enjoy the foods you love too!

5. Dieting not eating: Over the past few decades, the billion-dollar diet industry has misled you. When you eat, you will not lose weight (long-term). Yeah, I know, that's controversial and is the topic for another post – but the fact remains that research has shown that only 2-3 per cent of people who lose weight on a diet can successfully hold the weight off in the long term.

You deprive yourself when you limit the consumption of food in any way by dieting. The mental deprivation comes from realizing that as soon as you know that everything you want more is not allowed – and finally give in and have it! The physical denial comes from knowing that you start eating it again as soon as you can eat it again (you come off the diet when you reach your goal) and the weight goes back straight on. Hypnosis will help you achieve healthy, positive and sustainable weight loss by modifying your food choices, eating habits and body image.

Melanie Johnson

Melanie Johnson

Chapter 4: Steps for Weight Loss

Losing weight with hypnosis works just like any other change with hypnosis will. However, it is important to understand the step by step process so that you know exactly what to expect during your weight loss journey with the support of hypnosis. In general, there are about seven steps that are involved with weight loss using hypnosis. The first step is when you decide to change; the second step involves your sessions; the third and fourth are your changed mindset and behaviors, the fifth step involves your regressions, the sixth is your management routines, and the seventh is your lasting change. To give you a better idea of what each of these parts of your journey looks like, let's explore them in greater detail below.

In your first step toward achieving weight loss with hypnosis, you have decided that you desire change and that you are willing to try hypnosis as a way to change your approach to weight loss. At this point, you are aware of the fact that you want to lose weight, and you have been shown the possibility of losing weight through hypnosis. This is likely the stage you are in right now as you begin reading this very book. You may find yourself feeling curious, open to trying something new, and a little bit skeptical as to whether or not this is actually going to work for you. You may also be feeling frustrated, overwhelmed, or even defeated by the lack of success you have seen using other weight loss methods, which may be what lead you to seek out hypnosis in the first place. At this step, the most useful thing you can do is practice keeping an open and curious mind, as this is how you can set yourself up for success when it comes to your actual hypnosis sessions.

Your sessions account for stage two of the process. Technically, you are going to move from stage two through to stage five several times over before you officially move into stage six. Your sessions are the stage where you actually engage in hypnosis, nothing more and nothing less. During your sessions, you need to maintain your open mind and stay focused on how hypnosis can help you. If you are struggling to stay open-minded or are still skeptical about how this might work, you can consider switching from absolute confidence that it will help to have curiosity about how it might help instead.

Following your sessions, you are first going to experience a changed mindset. This is where you start to feel far more confident in your ability to lose weight and in your ability to keep the weight off. At first, your mindset may still be shadowed by doubt, but as you continue to use hypnosis and see your results, you will realize that it is entirely possible for you to create success with hypnosis. As these pieces of evidence start to show up in your own life, you will find your hypnosis sessions becoming even more powerful and even more successful.

In addition to a changed mindset, you are going to start to see changed behaviors. They may be smaller at first, but you will find that they increase over time until they reach the point where your behaviors reflect exactly the lifestyle you have been aiming to have. The best part about these changed behaviors is that they will not feel forced, nor will they feel like you have had to encourage yourself to get here: your changed mindset will make these changed behaviors incredibly easy for you to choose. As you continue working on your hypnosis and experiencing your changed mind, you will find that your behavioral changes grow more significant and more effortless every single time.

Following your hypnosis and your experiences with changed mindset and behaviors, you are likely going to experience regression periods. Regression periods are characterized by periods of time where you begin to engage in your old mindset and behavior once again. This happens because you have experienced this old mindset and behavioral patterns so many times over that they continue to have deep roots in your subconscious mind. The more you uproot them and reinforce your new behaviors with consistent hypnosis sessions, the more success you will have in eliminating these old behaviors and replacing them entirely with new ones. Anytime you experience the beginning of a regression period; you should set aside some time to engage in a hypnosis session to help you shift your mindset back into the state that you want and need it to be in.

Your management routines account for the sixth step, and they come into place after you have effectively experienced significant and lasting change from your hypnosis practices. At this point, you are not going to need to schedule as frequent of hypnosis sessions because you are experiencing such significant changes in your mindset. However, you may still want to do hypnosis sessions on a fairly consistent basis to ensure that your mindset remains changed and that you do not revert into old patterns. Sometimes, it can take up to 3-6 months or longer with these consistent management routine hypnosis sessions to maintain your changes and prevent you from experiencing a significant regression in your mindset and behavior.

The final step in your hypnosis journey is going to be the step where you come upon lasting changes. At this point, you are unlikely to need to schedule hypnosis sessions any longer. You should not need to rely on hypnosis at all to change your mindset because you have experienced such significant changes already, and you no longer find yourself regressing into old behaviors. With that being said, you may find that from time to time, you need to have a hypnosis session just to maintain your changes, particularly when an unexpected trigger may arise that may cause you to want to regress your behaviors. These unexpected changes can happen for years following your successful changes, so staying on top of them and relying on your healthy coping method of hypnosis is important as it will prevent you from experiencing a significant regression later in life.

Melanie Johnson

Chapter 5: Attract Wealth and Success

At this moment in time, there is nothing - nothing more important for you to do except to relax physically and mentally more and more. From this moment on, each and every breath will just help you to feel more relaxed. Each and every breath will help you to feel and to be calmer and calmer. And from this moment on, any sound outside this room will not affect or disturb you in any way. In fact, any sound outside this room will just help you to feel more relaxed. Any normal or outside noises will just help you to feel and just help you to be calmer and calmer.

Just listening now to the sound of my voice. The sound of my voice is just helping engage you into deeper relaxation. And in a few moments, I will count from ten down to one. With each and every number that I count from ten down to one, you'll you feel and just become more and more relaxed. With each and every number that I count from ten down to one, you'll just feel and you'll just become calmer and calmer. With each and every number that I count from ten down to one, you'll just drift deeper and deeper into relaxation. Not because I say so, but because it's the nature of the human mind to enjoy and to enjoy these wonderful levels of physical and mental relaxation absolutely. It really does feels good relaxing physically and it really does feel good just relaxing mentally more and more.

So, ten, beginning now to relax just more and more with every breath.

Nine each breathe just helping you to feel more and more relaxed. Each and every breath just helping you to be calmer and calmer. Each breath is helping you to drift deeper and deeper...and relax...

Eight and all muscles in your body from the top of your head down to your muscles in your feet feel and become more relaxed now.

And seven, as the muscles in your body feel and become more and more relaxed; your mind becomes just calmer and calmer.

And six, your mind and your body continue to become more and more relaxed. Continue to become just calmer and calmer.

Five, drifting deeper and deeper relaxed. Just feeling and just becoming calmer and calmer.

And five drifts into four and you drift deeper and deeper into relaxation.

Three, just enjoying this wonderful feeling, just enjoying this wonderful feeling of mental relaxation.

Two, calmer and more relaxed and becoming calm and just feeling more relaxed with each and every passing moment.

And one, and from this moment on, each and every breath you exhale just helps you to feel just helps you to be more relaxed. From this moment on, each and every breath just helps you to feel, and just helps you to be calmer and calmer. And from this moment on, with each and every day and hour that passes by you really are doing those things which you know inside your mind will bring success and will bring wealth into your life.

And one of the wonderful things about success, success is everywhere. You live and see that success. Success reveals itself everywhere you go. If you think about it, the computer that you're using is success. The pens that you write with are success. The car that you may drive is success. Success is revealed everywhere that you go. Each and every time you switch on a light that is success. And that success started with an idea, a wonderful idea that led to light being everywhere that you go, and ideas are powerful when they're acted upon. Ideas are almost like seeds and not acting on an idea it's just like having a seed in your hand. That seed in your hand is useless. That seed with that full potential to grow will not grow in your hand.

Just like an idea in your mind will not grow without action. That seed needs to be planted. That seed needs to be watered. That seed need action. And once the action is put into place that seed grows. That seed could begin to grow stronger and stronger and stronger just like an idea. An idea in your mind with action. That idea can simply grow and can become stronger and stronger and stronger. Life really is a wonderful fantastic journey. It's a wonderful journey where you can bring some wonderful things into your life. Life can give you what you want and as you receive life becomes a wonderful fantastic journey.

And every single day you're on this journey, every single day that passes by you get control you get to decide where this journey that you're on leads because one of the wonderful things about today is that all you can control is today. Today really is your past and future. And today is your future's past. So what things are you going to do today to bring success, to bring wealth into your life. Every single day you have decisions to make, choices to make. And those decisions, those choices that you make every single day will have an effect on your future. Today is really just your future's past. Just like today is your past's future. So what do you want your future to be? How do you want your future to pan out? What things do you want in your life? Just spend a few moments now thinking about those things.

Spend a few moments thinking what you want in your life. And I will give you a few moments as you think about those things now.

And as you think about those things, every part of you feels and just becomes more motivated now to bring those things into your life. As you think about those things, each and every part of you just feels and just becomes more and more determined to bring those things into your life. With every passing moment now, with every passing second of your life you really do believe more and more that you're going to bring those things into your life because in every single day now that passes by you're doing things and you're taking action. Turning those ideas into reality.

Success comes from doing - wealth comes from doing. You don't become successful; you don't become wealthy by just thinking about being successful by just thinking about being wealthy. Successful people become successful by doing things, by taking action. Wealthy people become wealthy by doing things and by taking action. And every single day, you're taking action. Every single day, you're making decisions and you're reaching your dreams. Every single day you're motivated, you're determined and you have a wonderful belief that you are going to bring those things into your life.

Each day, you're moving towards your goals. You're moving towards your dreams. You're moving towards wealth because every single day the decisions that you make move you towards where you want to be. Decisions and actions move you towards what you want or move you away from what you want. Isn't that how simple life can really be? A simple equation. Successful people in life are the doers. The successful people in life are people that take action. The successful people do more things; take more action than the people who only want to be successful.

Wealthy people take more action; make more decisions than people who don't have wealth in their lives. And with every single day now you're taking action, you can think of action, you can think of decisions of life being almost like a balance scale. And you can imagine on one side of the scale is success and wealth. The other side of the scale is being unsuccessful and even being poor.

With every single day that passes by, you have decisions to make whether to watch that TV program, deciding to stay in bed for another hour instead of doing something that you know would bring success into your life as putting weight to the side of being unsuccessful. Or by switching the TV off by getting out of bed and taking action. Doing something that you know will bring success into your life as putting weight onto that side of the scale of success; onto that side of wealth.

And with every single day now that passes you're using your time correctly. You're using your time wisely. Life really is one big clock that constantly is ticking by, you cannot speed time up. You cannot slow time down. It's constantly ticking by. Tick tock. Tick tock. And things that you do each day will predetermine what will future will be. One of the wonderful things about time is everybody has the same amount of time.

Every single day starts the same amount of time. Every day you have 24hours to use. You have 1,440 minutes to use. And you have 86,400 seconds every single day. And every single day, things that you do with that time is either putting weight on that side of success and wealth or putting weight on that side of unsuccessfulness, being poor and every day you really are now making the right decisions. You're making the right decisions. You're putting that weight towards success. You're putting that weight on the side of wealth. And wealth and success because of that is really coming into your life. You really are on a wonderful fantastic journey.

It's also important to realize on this journey, you will do things and you will fail. You may try something and it might not go correctly. And in a way that could be life testing you, seeing how much you really want this. If you do something and fail and quit, then you didn't want it bad enough. Many of the inventions if not all of the inventions we see around us came about by many mistakes by many so called famous. Thomas Edison, a report of one says how it felt to fail 9,999 times to which Mr. Edison replied "I never failed once. I found 9,999 things which didn't work. And for those 9,999 things which didn't work, I found one thing that did work by doing something and realizing what didn't work.

Melanie Johnson

You can change the approach. You can do something differently. It was all part of that wonderful journey and being on that wonderful journey brought that invention to success. That invention that's all around us each time you switch on a light. That light was first just an idea. An idea in someone's mind. And that wonderful idea is now everywhere because of action. Because of the decision of using time correctly.

Melanie Johnson

Chapter 6: Types of Food to Avoid and Why

There are lots of foods that do not help with your chronic inflammation.

Alcohol overworks your liver. The anti-inflammatory advises that you drink as little alcohol as possible. This prevents your liver from having to work overtime which causes internal inflammation.

Sugar is a tricky product to avoid because it is usually in everything that we eat! When you eat sugar, it releases cytokines or proteins in your body that trigger inflammation. High Fructose syrup is a very important word to look out for! Junk food like cookies and sodas are very important to limit.

Aspartame is an FDA-approved product that is an artificial sweetener that gives you no nutrients in your body. Many people react negatively to it. If your body reacts negatively towards this product, it will cause inflammation since your body recognizes it as a foreign product. When you are looking for sugar in products that you are buying, be sure to watch out for aspartame. Good luck since it is in over 4,000 products!

White flour is found in white potatoes and rice, bread, crackers and rolls, French fries and instant mash potatoes. When you eat white flour products, they release advanced glycation. End products in these can cause inflammation. To prevent inflammation, it is best to avoid these products.

Processed foods are foods that are already prepared and require limited cooking. Foods in this category include soups and sauces in cans, pre-cooked freezer meat, microwavable dinners, and deli meat. These foods typically contain a lot of sugar, salt, and trans-fats.

Omega-6 fatty acids are a necessity of your body to go through the natural growth and development cycle. In order for the natural growth and development cycle to be successful, your body needs a normal balance of fatty acids that are omega-3 and omega-6. When you eat too much omega-6 fatty acids, it throws your balance off and triggers inflammation in your body. The issue is that omega-6 fatty acids are found everywhere! They are in lots of salad dressings, mayonnaise, and most cooking oils. A major way to avoid omega-6 is to give up fried food which is found in lots of fast food.

Mono-sodium glutamate (MSG) is typically found in soup mixes, salad dressings, deli meats in Asian Foods, and soy sauce. This additive affects your liver's health and causes chronic inflammation. Try to avoid it.

Trans fats and partially hydrogenated oils are the same things. Trans fats raise your LDL cholesterol (low-density lipoprotein cholesterol) levels. Too much LDL cholesterol can cause inflammation of your heart and heart disease. Do not buy it at all if you want to remain inflammation free.

Saturated fats can cause heart disease and make your arthritis inflammation worse! Saturated fats cause inflammation of your fat tissue. Guess what the biggest sources of saturated fats are? It is pizza and cheese! You can also get saturated fats from red meat. If you must have meat, choose the leanest cuts like sirloin, loin or ground. Then trim off as much fat as you can before cooking. Also, for the cheese and dairy lovers, go for low-fat dairy.

Salt can cause tissue inflammation! It is found in lots of junk food and many people tend to over salt their food. When you are cooking, try to use other herbs and spices besides salt to season your food and watch your inflammation go down.

Gluten is found in whole grains like barley, rye, wheat or casein. It is also found in some dairy products. For those that have arthritis, eliminating gluten can be helpful. If you notice that when you eat gluten, you have inflammation and pain, you could also be at risk for celiac disease. Once you give up gluten, you can determine if it is a trigger for your inflammation. Then proceed based on your results. If gluten does not bother you, feel free to eat whole grains.

Melanie Johnson

Chapter 7: __come gestire I pasti della tua giornata:__ __colazione, pranzo e cena__

Here's a little secret. Exercise causes inflammation. Hear me out. When you do a tough workout, your body initiates acute inflammation to repair and rebuild your cells. However, this type of acute inflammation is good in the short-term which results in helping you improve chronic inflammation. If you notice that you are constantly tired after doing an intense workout, this point to you potentially having chronic inflammation. You may want to consider altering your exercise routine, doing shorter periods or change your workout to see if your chronic inflammation persists or not. The most important thing when working out is to make sure that you are recovering between your workouts in order to get the most out of your exercise regimen.

Some types of exercises that are really good to couple with your anti-inflammatory diet and boot the diet's benefits are yoga, walking or hiking.

Yoga is so great at fighting inflammation because of the deep breathing. When oxygen goes to your cells, it repairs them quickly and helps with chronic inflammation. The deep breathing associated with doing yoga is an excellent inflammation buster. There are three poses that are very helpful with combating inflammation, but any restorative yoga pose is beneficial to preventing inflammation.

Half lord of the fish is the first pose. This reduces chronic inflammation by cleaning the digestive system and organs associated with your intestines. To start, you find a comfortable place to sit and extend both of your legs. You put the right foot outside the left quad as far as possible. Then you put your foot on the left side outside the hip on your right side. Then you want to swing the elbow on your left side of your body to the knee on the right side of your body. Try to get it as far as the outside of your right knee as you can. You can use the hand on your right side as extra support. Now in this pose, you want to be mindful of your back. Make sure that you are listening to your spine by drawing the crown of your head to the sky. You want to try this on both sides and then hold 5-7 deeps breaths on each side.

Another very popular yoga poses to battle chronic inflammation is called the child's pose. You first want to get comfortable by doing the tabletop pose which is simply putting your shoulders and your wrist forwards then putting your hips over your knees. You want to bring your big toes as close as possible. Then you want to sit on your hip gently. This allows the Torso to rest between your knees with your arms stretched out in front of you as far as possible. Hold for 5 to 7 breaths on each side as well.

Do not underestimate walking's power to fight inflammation. Walking is so great at reducing inflammation because it sends fresh oxygen and blood throughout your body. Immersing yourself in nature helps lower your cortisol stress response, that is very important in reducing inflammation. Overall, no matter, what exercise you do, it is important to listen to your body. It will tell you when it had enough or if you should keep going.

Melanie Johnson

After your workout, it is important to make sure that you are eating an anti-inflammatory meal with foods that will help you recover after doing a workout. After working out, if you can reduce inflammation, it will help prevent the soreness that comes up sometimes after your workout called delayed onset muscle soreness or DOMS. Eating about 30 to 60 minutes after you cool down will help replace the glycogen stores that will help you heal quickly. Some great foods to eat after working out would be black beans because they help repair muscle damage. Leafy greens like spinach, Brussel sprouts, kale, broccoli are another good food to aid in your post-workout recovery. They help you hydrate without causing a spike in sugar. If you are pushed for time and do not have time to make a meal, a quick and easy post-workout snack is to add spices to yogurt or in a post-workout smoothie like turmeric, ginger or cinnamon.

Breakfast

To make sure you get all your vegetables, you can eat a savory, vegetable-based breakfast so that you get what you need. Really, vegetables are great to have at any time of day because they help stabilize our mood, especially if you get stressed throughout the day.

Avoid oranges at breakfast because it can cause stomach irritation which can lead to inflammation.

Avoid zucchini for breakfast because it has a diuretic effect and can cause dehydration if you haven't drunk anything yet for the morning.

The best time to eat apples is at breakfast because of the pectin in the apple's skin. Pectin helps your intestines remove toxic things from your body. Apples are horrible at dinnertime because apples increase stomach acid which can lead to discomfort.

Tomatoes are great to have at breakfast because the type of acid found in tomatoes can help your digestive processes and regulate the functions of your stomach and pancreas.

The best time to have potatoes is at breakfast because it lowers our blood cholesterol level and it is also rich in minerals that your body needs to power you throughout the day.

A fiber-packed bowl of oatmeal topped with peanut butter and berries sets the tone for the day for your digestive tract.

Also, have chocolate for breakfast. Sounds counterintuitive, but when you have dark chocolate in the morning, it protects your skin against sun rays, and it gives you all day to burn the calories off.

Lunch

The best time to eat carbohydrates is during and after physical activity because this is when your body can best handle them. You may want to eat a lower amount of carbs daily if you are sedentary most of the time to prevent weight gain.

The best time to eat meat is at lunchtime. It helps to reduce fatigue by giving a steady flow of nutrients throughout the rest of the day. It also takes meat for about 5 hours to digest. By eating it at lunch, you give your body ample time to digest the meat. However, if you eat meat at dinner, be sure to eat it early enough before you go to bed so your food can be digested.

Another great thing to eat at lunch is raw nuts because it helps your body with the fatty acids that are omega 3. Since nuts have a high-calorie count and fat count, if you eat them for dinner, you can gain unwanted weight.

Pasta is best to have for breakfast and lunch so your body can digest the food throughout the rest of the day.

The best time to have rice is at lunch as it is high in carbohydrates and can help you stay energized. If you eat rice at dinner, then it could potentially lead to weight gain.

Dinner

Because potatoes are two to three times higher in calories than other vegetables, you do not want to have them for dinner.

Tomatoes at dinnertime can cause swelling.

For dinner, it is great to have something spicy to aid in digestion, but if you have an unfavorable reaction, please avoid it.

Melanie Johnson

Chapter 8: Techniques to Reach Your Ideal Weight

Techniques to lose weight

1. Drink water!

Studies show that adding more water to your daily diet helps you lose weight; you naturally reduce the amount of food you eat.

Replace sweetened drinks or sugary drinks.

We can never repeat it enough, the human body needs 1.5l of water per day, sodas and other fruit juices do not enter this daily 1.5l. Not only are these sugary drinks sources of empty calories, but they fuel your appetite for sugar and sweet tastes.

2. Eat full

A balanced diet based on whole foods can naturally help stabilize your weight.

Choose good fats, complex carbohydrates (wholegrain pasta, wholegrain rice, wholegrain bread, sweet potatoes, quinoa, and buckwheat) and lean proteins (white meats, vegetable proteins) to benefit from good nutritional intakes while contributing to your satiety.

Plant fibers are particularly appreciated because they also contribute to satiety and a better intestinal balance... always this question of balance.

3. Limit your exposure to additives

Certain components that you find daily in your diet contribute to weight gain, or prevent weight loss.

These chemicals act as endocrine disruptors and change the response of your hormonal system to the hunger and envy signals normally sent by your brain.

Beware of BPA (Bisphenol A - it is found in many plastics and cans -, perfluorooctanoic acid - present in many cleaning and non-stick products - pesticides of course, phthalates - PVC, cosmetics, clothing, toys- difficult to track because they are found everywhere.

Open your eyes, learn, start to keep them away from your consumption, these endocrine disruptors are more and more identified as responsible for many cancers, too frequent fertility problems or early puberty in children.

4. Learn to manage your stress

Stress is a factor in weight gain for two reasons:

Melanie Johnson

Under stress, the body increases its secretion of cortisol (stress hormone) . When these hormones are produced in too large quantities, the body goes into fat storage mode and becomes more efficient at storing future fat!

The second reason that stress makes us gain weight is emotional. In times of stress, you will seek comfort, and it is very often found in food ... and unfortunately not the one that is good for you but rather fatty foods, sugars, and especially rich in empty calories.

So not only are we more attracted to high-calorie foods when we are stressed, but our bodies are also more efficient at turning them into fat

Some tips to reduce stress (through regular practice):

- Yoga

- Physical practice

- Meditation

- Music (that you play or listen to while being carried)
- Deep breathing
- Reading

5. Eat consciously

When you eat, try to slow down and be present at your meal. I know it is not always obvious, and it may even seem absurd. But experience it.

Sit down, take a deep breath, and take the time to chew each bite (ideally, chew each bite for 30 seconds, saliva contains enzymes that facilitate digestion and absorption of food), identify the tastes on your plate. By taking the time to be present at your meal, naturally your quantities will decrease.

6. Breakfast

Melanie Johnson

A habit that everyone who has successfully lost weight and stabilized has had is to eat breakfast each morning. I know there is a lot of talk about intermittent fasting at the moment, I also practice it and I cannot dispute its effectiveness.

However, intermittent fasting is effective if lunch time is not expected as release. If you are in the process of losing weight, you absolutely have to avoid the situations that will lead to creating cravings (taking fast sugars or a badly managed fast) because following a cravings is to jump on any food that will quench your hunger, often in much more than you need.

Practice the intermittent youngster to compensate for an excess the day before for example, hydrate yourself all morning to eliminate and put your intestines a few hours at rest.

But each morning, choose a hearty, nutritious and low-sugar breakfast that will guarantee your energy intake necessary to start the day: whole meal bread, a hot drink, a little butter or coconut or linseed oil in a salad fruit, an egg.

Eat breakfast within an hour of waking up.

7. Don't skip meals

If you are trying to lose weight, make sure you are not overly hungry between meals. As I just mentioned, if you are too hungry, you are more likely to binge on the foods you are trying to eat limited. Not only are you more likely to make an impulsive eating decision, but you will eat a lot more than usual.

Take 3 meals a day, choose a light meal in the evening, do not hesitate to provide yourself with a snack in the afternoon if you dine a little late, and find solutions to avoid cravings at any time.

8. Cook at home

I know it is not always easy. If you are not used to cooking, the idea of cooking is exhausting in advance. However, preparing your own meals is the best way to control what you eat, limit industrial food, choose the right fats and in the right amount. It's also a good way to get flavor.

There are more and more vegetables already cut, pre-cooked, or quick frozen vegetables to prepare. A salad of small tomatoes, feta cheese, spinach leaves, tapenade sandwiches, sunflower seeds and olive oil for example is super quick to prepare and delicious in summer.

Make the experience by starting by preparing small simple and fast dishes, you will be able to taste it.

9. Sleep

Lacking sleep, going to bed late, being a victim of insomnia eventually disrupt your circadian rhythm, which unfortunately has the effect of increasing inflammatory states in your body, inflammatory states conducive to weight gain.

Sleep deprivation also causes your body to produce more ghrelin, a hormone that activates the hunger signal. This hormone, set on the circadian cycle, takes action upon awakening. The less you sleep, the more you stay awake, the more it will send the brain the signal to feed this constantly active body.

Melanie Johnson

A minimum of 7 hours of sleep per night is now recommended.

Some tips for sleeping well:

No electronic device (tablet, TV, telephone, Wi-Fi) in the bedroom

Eliminate blue lights and your field of vision

Cut the screens ideally 2 hours before bed

Read, it's very enriching intellectually, but also very soporific at night!

Dine light

Practice if you like gentle yoga (yoga nidra), some breathing exercises, such as heart coherence

Fall asleep at regular hours

10. Have regular physical practice

Melanie Johnson

Exercise helps relieve stress, burn calories, and give your metabolism an energy resource even when you're not training.

By practicing physical activity, you secrete serotonin, an important neurotransmitter in the central nervous system and especially in the synapses of the areas responsible for emotional activity. Serotonin deficiency creates emotional instability and is often equated with depression. Conversely, regular production of serotonin contributes to your emotional balance and well-being.

Make sure you consume some protein after your sport (almonds, walnuts, fresh fruit smoothies and chia seeds, oatmeal, almond milk and dried fruits, small homemade muffin -prepared with whole meal flour).

Melanie Johnson

Chapter 9: 6 Major steps to lose weight

Obesity contributes to many health problems like diabetes and hypertension. Weight loss of as little as 5% brings big benefits! Here are some steps to help you get started.

STEP 1: SET A REALISTIC GOAL

It can be difficult to navigate among concepts such as ideal weight, healthy weight and body mass index (BMI). Here is some information about it.

A priori, the concept of ideal weight is used in the medical community. It is the result of a calculation that can be performed using several different formulas that take into account the sex of the person, his size, and sometimes his age.

Melanie Johnson

A person's healthy weight is often established based on BMI. This tool allows you to calculate, by height, the weight range associated with optimal health. The further you go from this interval, the higher the risk of developing health problems. The BMI results from a very simple calculation: we take the weight of an individual (in kilograms) and divide it by the square of their height (in meters). Several factors such as age, gender, inheritance and bone structure are not taken into account. A normal BMI is usually between 18.5 and 25.

So do not hesitate to consult a nutritionist before undertaking a dietary change or weight loss. Also, if you have a health problem and are taking medication, talk to the pharmacist before changing your habits.

Already, not gaining weight is a victory in itself! It is better to set yourself a realistic goal and highlight your victories rather than aim for a great loss of weight and then be disappointed not to achieve it. It is better to adopt healthy habits and modify your diet in the long term than to aim for a number on the scale.

STEP 2: DEFINE YOUR MOTIVATIONS

It is not always easy to get motivated to change our habits, including eating habits. To maintain your motivation, it is important to be clear about the reasons why you are losing weight or changing your diet. Make a list of your motivations and post it in certain strategic places. This will help you always to keep them in mind.

STEP 3: THINK STRATEGIES

Melanie Johnson

When you want to reach a goal, you have to think of concrete ways to reach it and keep it in the long term in order to maintain the desired weight. Forget the "miracle regimes" focused on deprivation. The saying that you have to suffer to lose weight is false. This belief may not lead you to the desired results.

To achieve your goals, you should adopt this winning combination: modify your diet and increase your level of physical activity. Here are some examples of strategies that really work:

Eat a diet low in fat and sugar.

Eliminate processed foods from your diet.

Increase your intake of fruits, vegetables and other high-fiber foods.

Add more physical activity to your routine. Exercise 30 to 60 minutes a day, at least 5 days a week. Start slowly and gradually increase the intensity.

STEP 4: BUILD YOUR RESOURCE LIST

There are probably more resources available to help you than you think. Ask your doctor or pharmacist about the right resources to guide you: nutritionist, doctor, kinesiology, etc.

STEP 5: WRITE YOUR ACTION PLAN

Once you have set your goal and clarified your motivations, your strategies and your resources, it would be good to record all this information in a document that will serve as your action plan.

STEP 6: TAKE ACTION!

Melanie Johnson

That's it! Now that you are well prepared, it is time to act. Change your habits quietly or faster. You decide. But above all, highlight your victories and do not lose sight of your primary motivations.

In conclusion, it is easy to make good resolutions ... Maintaining them is a different story. We wish you success, and remember that when it comes to health decisions, your pharmacist is always there to support and encourage you!

Melanie Johnson

Chapter 10: Overcoming Negative Habits

Fortunately, most of our days have a sort of "groove." Actions in a plan that you perform with little thought are performed almost automatically. Otherwise, our lives become tediously complicated, and we spend a lot of time figuring out how to tie our shoes, prepare our meals, go to work, and more. In this way, we can carry out our daily routines with almost no thought and focus our attention on more demanding activities. Repetitive work in life becomes a habit.

Habits can also be undesirable, and these grooves are deeply rooted in today's patterns. They are against us because they waste our time. For example, if you know that you have a limited amount of time to get to work after waking up in the morning, you'll notice that in the middle of breakfast you'll find the morning paper at the table, pick it up, and usually spend the next hour studying. Spend In the daily news, you could spend a good deal of the rest of your time explaining delays or looking for new jobs.

By the way, we call them "desired" or "undesired" rather than "good" or "bad." The words "good" and "bad" have moral implications. These mean certain decisions. In the example cited in the paragraph above, reading a newspaper is not morally "bad," but not desirable at this time.

The terms "desired" and "undesirable" are the terms "ego," meaning self-determination, not decisions made externally. As with psychoanalysis, our goal is to push material from the "conscience" camp into the "ego" realm.

In many cases, you may even say that removing unnecessary habits requires more than a simple choice. You may want to discard your habits consciously, but fulfilling a wish is a very different matter. There are several reasons for this. First, habits are inherent in their definition and are deeply rooted in their behavior, so they are reflected without thinking. Just thinking "I don't do" does not necessarily affect us deep enough to stop unwanted behavior.

The longer the habit we have with us, the more often we do it, the more secure it will be, and the harder it will be to wipe it off. Please quit overeating. It is not uncommon to start eating without knowing it when already taken a full meal or when absorbed in conversation or work. Such behaviors are driven into individual behavioral patterns dozens of times a day, daily, and over ten years, actually becoming a second cortex that is as natural as breathing (ironically, overcoming eating habits are becoming increasingly difficult for people).

Such habits have physical-neurologic-foundation. The neural pathways in our body can be compared to unpaved roads. This road is smooth before vehicles drive on dirt roads. When a car first rides on the road, its tires leave marks, but the ruts are flat. Rain and wind can easily pass by and smooth the road again. However, after 100 rides with deeper and deeper tires, rain and wind make little impression on the deep ruts. They stay there.

The same applies to people. To expand the metaphor a little, we were born with a smooth street in our heads. When a young child first buttons a jacket or ties a shoe, the effort is tedious, clumsy, and frustrating. More trials are needed until the child gets the hang of it, and a successful move becomes a behavioral pattern.

From a physiological point of view, these movement instructions travel along nerve paths to the muscles and back again. The message is sent to the central nervous system along an afferent pathway. The "I want to lift my legs" impulse continues in the efferent pathway from the central nervous system to my muscles: "Raise my legs." After a while, such messages are automatically enriched by countless repetitions and automatically sent at electrical speed.

Return to the car and the street. Suppose the car decides to avoid a worn groove and take a new path. What's going on the car will go straight back into the old ditch. Like people trying to get out of old habits, they tend to revert to old habits.

Still, we haven't developed any unwanted habits. We learn them, and we can rewind the learning. It can be unconditional. And here, self-hypnosis takes place, pushing the individual out of the established habit gap in a smooth manner of new behavior.

The advantage it offers compared to simple willpower trial and error results from an increase in the state of consciousness that characterizes the state of self-hypnosis. As a neurological phenomenon in itself, this elevated state of consciousness appears to elevate the individual over behavioral patterns. A further extension of the unpaved road analogy is that the hovercraft slides a few centimeters above the road, over a rut or habit. Regardless of the habit of working, the implementation process is the same. Only the verbal implant and the image below are different. To encapsulate the induction process, count one, for one thing, two for two things and count three for three things:

1. Please raise your eyes as high as possible.

2. Still staring, slowly close your eyes and take a deep breath.

3. Exhale, relax your eyes, and float your body. Then, if time permits, spend a little more time and introduce yourself to the most comfortable, calm, and pleasant place in your imagination.

Now, when you float deep inside the resting chair, you will feel a little away from your body. It's another matter, so you can give her instructions on how to behave.

Melanie Johnson

At this point, the specific purpose of self-hypnosis determines the expression and image content of the syllogism. This strategy can help overcome the habit of overeating.

Overall, we are a country boasting abundant food. Most of us (with the blatant and lamentable exception) have enough money to make sure we are comfortably overeating. As a result, many of us get obese. So, the weight loss business is a big industry. Tablet makers, diet developers, and exercise studios will not confuse customers who want to lose weight.

It is said that every fat person who has a hard time escaping has lost weight. Unfortunately, too often, the lean man spends his life, nevertheless never succeeding in his escape. Despite the image of a funny fat man, everyone rarely enjoys being overweight-most people become unhappy, rarely so confident and less than confident and ruining their lives. Obesity seems to creep on only some of us, and by the time we notice it, it is a painful habit to overeat or eat, like the excess weight itself.

Self-hypnosis can help this lean man release his bond of "too hard" and start a new life.

Dr. Roger Bernhardt, while mentioning one of his overweight patients, said that "I brought the patient to the hospital for about a year and a half ago. She went to many doctors to cut back. She said she was rarely leaving home because she was extremely obese; she was relaxing and avoiding people. She came in for £ 380. I started Trans in my first session. She continued on a diet and focused on telling her she would like people when she lost weight. She came for the first three or four sessions each week, after which I started teaching her self-hypnosis. Now, this woman lost a total of £ 150, but beyond that, she became another person. She was virtually introverted and rarely came out of her home. She dared to do a part-time job in cosmetics. She hosts a party to show off her cosmetics and hypnotizes herself before the party. She became the state's second-largest saleswoman and earned tens of thousands of dollars."

Simply put, here are the therapies you should use when using self-hypnosis for weight management. After provoking self-hypnosis, mentally recite the syllogism. "I need my body alive. To the extent I want to live, I protect my body just as I protect it."

In the case of a tie mate picture, one can imagine himself in two situations where he is likely to overeat:

between meals and at the dining table. With his eyes closed, he imagines a movie screen on the wall. He is on the screen himself, in every situation he finds when he is reading, chatting with others, watching TV, or having trouble calorie counting.

Instead of reaching for popcorn, potato chips, or peanuts as before, he is now simply focusing on the conversation, the television screen, or the printed page, perhaps except for a glass of water, and I congratulate you on being unfamiliar with anything at the table.

The second scene that catches your eye is the dining table. Do you tend to grab this second loaf? Instead, put your hand on your forehead and remember, "Protect my body." Looking at a cake, a loaf, a potato, or a cake raises the idea, "This is for someone. I'm good enough".

With the fork down, take a deep breath and be proud to help one-person flow through the body.

Then, imagine a very simple and effective exercise method that simply puts your hand on the edge of the table and pushes it. Better yet, stand up from the chair and leave the table at this point.

Here's another image I'd recommend to a self-hypnotist. If you introduce yourself to the screen of this fictional movie, you will find yourself slim. Give yourself the ideal line that you want to see to others. Cut the abdomen and waistline to the desired ratio. Take an imaginary black pencil, sketch the entire picture, and make the lines sharp and solid. Hold photo because you can keep this slender picture, you can lose weight.

Then get out of your hypnosis and repeat it regularly every few hours. Exercise is especially useful during the temptation to be used as a comfortable, calorie-free substitute for fatty snacks or as an additional serving with meals. It would be an excellent time to prepare it just before dinner.

Melanie Johnson

Chapter 11: Mindful Eating Habits

Understanding Mindful Eating

There are various scopes of cautious eating techniques, some of them established in Zen and different kinds of Buddhism, others connected to yoga. Here, we are taking a simple technique.

My careful eating procedure is figuring out how to be cautious. Rather than eating carelessly, putting nourishment unknowingly in your mouth, not so much tasting the sustenance you eat, you see your thoughts, and feelings.

• Learn to be cautious: why you want to eat, and what emotions or requirements can trigger eating.

• What you eat, and whether it's solid.

• Look, smell, taste, feel the nourishment that you eat.

• How do you feel like when you taste it, how would you digest it, and go about your day?

• During and in the wake of eating, your sentiments.

• Where the nourishment originated from, who could have developed it, the amount it could have suffered before it was killed, regardless of whether it was naturally developed, the amount it was handled, the amount it was broiled or overcooked, and so on.

This is ability that you don't simply increase medium-term, a type of reflection. It takes practice, and there will be times when you neglect to eat mindfully, beginning, and halting. However, you can get generally excellent at this with exercise and consideration.

Mindful Eating Benefits

The upsides of eating mindfully are unimaginable and realizing these points of interest is fundamental as you think about the activity.

• When you're anxious, you find out how to eat and stop when you're plunking down.

• You find out how to taste nourishment and acknowledge great sustenance tastes.

• You start to see gradually that unfortunate nourishment isn't as scrumptious as you accepted, nor does it make you feel extremely pleasant.

• Because of the over three points, if you are overweight, you will regularly get more fit.

• You start arranging your nourishment and eating through the passionate issues you have. It requires somewhat more, yet it's basic.

• Social overeating can turn out to be less of an issue— you can eat mindfully while mingling, rehearsing, and not over-alimenting.

• You begin to appreciate the experience of eating more, and as an outcome, you will acknowledge life more when you are progressively present.

• It can transform into a custom of mindfulness that you anticipate.

• You learn for the day how nourishment impacts your disposition and vitality.

• You realize what fuel your training best with nourishment and you work and play.

Melanie Johnson

A Guide to Mindful Eating

Keeping up a contemporary, quick-paced way of life can leave a brief period to oblige your necessities. You are moving always starting with one thing then onto the next, not focusing on what your psyche or body truly needs. Rehearsing mindfulness can help you to comprehend those necessities.

When eating mindfulness is connected, it can help you recognize your examples and practices while simultaneously standing out to appetite and completion related to body signs.

Originating from the act of pressure decrease dependent on mindfulness, rehearsing mindfulness while eating can help you focus on the present minute instead of proceeding with ongoing and unacceptable propensities.

Careful eating is an approach to begin an internal looking course to help you become increasingly aware of your nourishment association and utilize that information to eat with joy.

The body conveys a great deal of information and information, so you can start settling on cognizant choices as opposed to falling into programmed — and regularly feeling driven — practices when you apply attention to the eating knowledge. You are better prepared to change your conduct once you become aware of these propensities.

Individuals that need to be cautious about sustenance and nourishment are asked to:

- Explore their inward knowledge about sustenance—different preferences

- Choose sustenance that please and support their bodies

- Accept explicit sustenance inclinations without judgment or self-analysis

- Practice familiarity with the indications of their bodies beginning to eat and quit eating.

General Principles of Mindful Eating

One methodology to careful eating depends on the core values given by Rebecca J. Frey, Ph.D., and Laura Jean Cataldo, RN: tune in to the internal craving and satiety signs of your body Identify private triggers for careless eating, for example, social weights, amazing sentiments, and explicit nourishments.

Here are some tips for getting you started.

• Start with one meal. It requires some investment to begin with any new propensity. It very well may be difficult to make cautious eating rehearses constantly. However, you can practice with one dinner or even a segment of a supper. Attempt to focus on appetite sign and sustenance choices before you start eating or sinking into the feelings of satiety toward the part of the arrangement—these are phenomenal approaches to begin a routine with regards to consideration.

• Remove view distractions place or turn off your phone in another space. Mood killers such the TV and PC and set away whatever else —, for example, books, magazines, and papers—that can divert you from eating. Give the feast before your complete consideration.

• Tune in your perspective when you start this activity, become aware of your attitude. Perceive that there is no right or off base method for eating, yet simply unmistakable degrees of eating background awareness. Focus your consideration on eating sensations. When you understand that your brain has meandered, take it delicately back to the eating knowledge.

• Draw in your senses with this activity. There are numerous approaches to explore. Attempt to investigate one nourishment thing utilizing every one of your faculties. When you put sustenance in your mouth, see the scents, surfaces, hues, and flavors. Attempt to see how the sustenance changes as you cautiously bite each nibble.

• Take as much time as necessary. Eating cautiously includes backing off, enabling your stomach related hormones to tell your mind that you are finished before eating excessively. It's a fabulous method to hinder your fork between chomps. Additionally, you will be better arranged to value your supper experience, especially in case you're with friends and family.

Rehearsing mindfulness in a bustling globe can be trying now and again; however, by knowing and applying these essential core values and techniques, you can discover approaches to settle your body all the more promptly. When you find out how much your association with nourishment can adjust to improve things, you will be charmingly astounded — and this can importantly affect your general prosperity and wellbeing.

Melanie Johnson

Formal dinners, be that as it may, will, in general, assume a lower priority about occupied ways of life for generally people. Rather, supper times are an opportunity to endeavor to do each million stuff in turn. Consider having meals at your work area or accepting your Instagram fix over breakfast to control through a task.

The issue with this is you are bound to be genuinely determined in your decisions about healthy eating and eat excessively on the off chance that you don't focus on the nourishment you devour or the way you eat it.

That is the place mindfulness goes in. You can apply similar plans to a yoga practice straight on your lunch plate". Cautious eating can enable you to tune in to the body's information of what, when, why, and the amount to eat," says Lynn Rossy, Ph.D., essayist of The

Melanie Johnson

Mindfulness-Based Eating Solution and the Center for Mindful Eating director. "Rather than relying upon another person (or an eating routine) to reveal to you how to eat, developing a minding association with your own body can achieve tremendous learning and change."

From the ranch to the fork — can help you conquer enthusiastic eating, make better nourishment choices, and even experience your suppers in a crisp and ideally better way. To make your next dinner mindful, pursue these measures.

The most effective method to Start Eating More Intentionally

Stage 1: Eat Before You Shop. We have all been there. You go with a rumbling stomach to the shop. You meander the passageways, and out of the blue, those power bars and microwaveable suppers start to look truly enticing. "When you're excessively ravenous, shopping will, in general, shut us off from our progressively talented goals of eating in a way that searches useful for the body," says Dr. Rossy. So, even if you feel the slightest craving or urge to eat, get a nutritious bite or a light meal before heading out. That way, your food choices will be made intentionally when you shop, as opposed to propelled by craving or an unexpected sugar crash in the blood.

Stage 2: Make Conscious Food Choices. When you truly start considering where your nourishment originates from, you're bound to pick sustenance that is better for you, the earth, and the people occupied with the expanding procedure portrays Meredith Klein, an astute cooking educator, and Pranaful's author. "When you're in the supermarket, focus on the nourishment source," Klein shows. "Hope to check whether it's something that has been created in this country or abroad and endeavors to know about pesticides that may have been exposed to or presented to people who were developing nourishment." If you can, make successive adventures to your neighborhood ranchers advertise, where most sustenance is developed locally, she recommends.

Stage 3: Enjoy the Preparation Process. "When you get ready sustenance, instead of looking at it as an errand or something you need to hustle through, value the process. You can take a great deal of pleasure in food shopping for items that you know will help you feel better and nourish your body.

Stage 4: "Simply eat". This is something we once in a while do, as simple as it sounds, "Simply eat." "Individuals regularly eat while doing different things — taking a gander at their telephones, TVs, PCs, and books, and mingling," claims Dr. Rossy. "While cautious eating can happen when you're doing other stuff, endeavor to' simply eat' at whatever point plausible." She includes that centering the nourishment you're eating without preoccupation can make you mindful of flavors you may never have taken note of. Yum!

Stage 5: Down Your Utensils. When you are done eating, immediately put your dishes and utensils away. This is a way of signaling to yourself that you are done eating (it tends to be much a bit tough to accept). "You're getting a charge out of each chomp that way, and you're focused on the nibble that is in your mouth right now as opposed to setting up the following one," Klein says.

Stage 6: Chew, Chew, Chew Your Food. Biting your sustenance is exceptionally fundamental and not only for, have you known, not to stun. "When we cautiously eat our sustenance, we help the body digest the nourishment all the more effectively and meet a greater amount of our dietary needs," says Dr. Rossy.

Melanie Johnson

Furthermore, no, we won't educate you how often you've eaten your sustenance. However, Dr. Rossy demonstrates biting until the nourishment is very much separated – which will most likely take more than a couple of quick eats.

Melanie Johnson

Melanie Johnson

Chapter 12: trucchi pratici per assumere meno calorie capitolo

For the greatest part, when we are speaking about losing weight and ensuring that we can get our health in the right order that we want, we will focus on the exercise and the diet. Both of these are important. One is going to ensure that we are able to lose weight and keep our hearts as strong as possible in the process and is known for helping to fight off a lot of the different diseases that are out there. But the other one will help to reduce weight and can ensure the body is getting the nutrients that it really needs as well.

However, there are a few other options that we are able to do that can make it easier to lose the weight and eat fewer calories overall, so that we can lose the weight without all of the stress. These are going to be so effective when it comes to reducing your own weight and can prevent some of the weight gains that we are worried about seeing in the future. Some of these are going to include:

Slow Down and Chew

We have to start slowing down when it is time to eat our meals. We need to give the brain some time to process what you are eating and to know when you have had enough to eat. When you chew the food all the way through, it is going to force you to slow down in your eating, and it is going to be associated back with a decreased amount of food that you take in. It can make you seem full faster and you will take on smaller portion sizes.

Melanie Johnson

How fast you are able to finish your meals can also have a big effect on your current weight. One review that was done on 23 observational studies found that the people who ate their meals a lot faster were more likely to gain weight than those who were the slower eaters. And fast eaters in these studies were also the ones who are more likely to be obese.

This is an easy thing to fix. You can set a timer and not allow yourself to eat faster than that at any time. You can also make it be set up so that you count how many times that you chew each bite, and then take a drink of water in between. This is going to be an easy way to help you to slow down and will make it easier to eat less at the meal.

Go with Smaller Plates

You will find that the typical food plate is a lot bigger than it used to be. This is a trend that is going to contribute to weight gain because using a smaller plate can help you to eat less as your portions are going to look a lot larger than they are. This is a good way to ensure that you are going to trick your mind about how much it is eating.

On the other hand, when you work with a plate that is a lot bigger, it is going to make a serving, even one that is bigger, look smaller. You will be more likely to add on more food and eat more than you should. This means that you can use this to your advantage. If you are going to eat a lot of healthy foods, go with the bigger plate, so you take on bigger portions of it and get more of that good stuff. But if you are going to eat foods that are not as healthy, then go ahead and go with the plates that are smaller.

Add in the Protein

Protein is going to have some powerful effects on appetite. It is able to help us increase our feelings of fullness, can help us to reduce your hunger, and will make it easier to eat fewer calories. This may be because protein is going to affect several hormones that play a role in hunger and fullness, including the ghrelin hormone.

There is one study that found when we increase our protein intake from 15 percent to 30 percent of our calories, it made it easier for participants to take in 441 fewer calories per day and then lose 11 pounds over a 12 week period on average, and this was all without intentionally restricting any of the other foods that the participants were eating.

A good way to use this is with your own meals. If you are eating a breakfast that is full of grains, for example, then switching to a meal that is higher in protein may be a good place to start. In one study, it found that obese and overweight women who had eggs as part of their breakfast were able to eat fewer calories at lunch compared to those women who at a breakfast that was based more on grains.

Eat the Fiber

Eating foods that are rich in fiber is another way for us to make sure that we increase our satiety, which is going to help us to feel fuller for a longer period of time. Studies are also showing us that one type of fiber, which is known as viscous fiber, is going to be really helpful when it comes to weight loss. This one is so good because it is able to increase the amount of fullness that we have, and it is able to reduce the foods that we intake.

Viscous fiber is going to form a gel when it comes in contact with water. This gel is going to increase some of the nutrient absorption time and it is going to slow down how the stomach is able to empty out as well.

Viscous fiber is something that we are able to find in foods that are planted, so we are going to find it in places like flax seeds, oranges, asparagus, Brussels sprouts, oat cereals, and beans as well. Here is also a weight loss supplement out right now that is known as glucomannan, and it is going to have a high amount of this viscous fiber as well.

Drink Water Often

Make sure that drinking enough water on a regular basis because this will help us to fill up our stomachs so that we eat less and lose weight. This is going to happen even more when we make sure to drink before a meal. There was one study in adults that found that drinking about 17 ounces of water about half an hour before a meal would reduce the amount of hunger that was felt and help lessen how many calories the individual was going to take in.

Those participants in this study who took the time to drink more water before their meals were able to lose 44 percent more weight over a period of three months compared to those who did not have the water before their meals. If you are able to replace some of the regular drinks that you like to have, which are loaded with calories, such as juice or soda, with water, it is possible that the weight loss that you are experiencing will be even higher.

Melanie Johnson

Keep the Portions Small

In addition to those bigger plates that we were talking about before, you will find that portion sizes have really seen an increase over the past few decades, especially when we go out to eat. These larger portions are going to encourage people to eat more and can be linked back to an increase in weight and obesity overall as well.

In fact, there was one study in adults that fond that when the appetizer with the dinner was doubled, it was able to increase the number of calories that were taken in by 30 percent. You will find that serving yourself just a little bit less could be enough to help you to eat fewer calories, and if it very unlikely that you would even notice the difference.

Melanie Johnson

Don't Eat Neat the TV

Paying more attention to what you are eating could help you to take in fewer calories overall. Those who eat while they are on the computer or watching a show could easily lose track of the amount they are eating. This is going to cause them to overeat as well. one review of 24 studies found that those who were distracted when they were eating their meals would eat about 10 percent more during that sitting than those who paid attention.

In addition, being absent-minded when it came to the meal would have a bigger influence on how much you took in later in the day. Those who were more distracted during a meal would eat 25 percent more calories at later meals than those who paid more attention. If you are eating meals while watching TV or using some kind of electronic device, you are likely to eat more without noticing. These are calories that will add up and can have a big impact on your weight over time.

Try to Avoid Stress and Sleep More

Now, if you are a parent, you probably read the thing above and started laughing. Sleeping well and avoiding all of the stress can seem almost impossible when you are a parent, and you have a bunch of things to keep track of for your children. And if your children are not sleeping through the night yet, getting that sleep that you need may seem almost impossible as well. This is also why a lot of parents are going to gain weight when taking care of their children and it is a good example of why we need to pay a bit more attention to our own sleeping styles to ensure that we get enough.

When it comes to your health, people are often going to neglect taking care of their stress or getting enough sleep. Both of these are going to have really powerful effects on your weight and your sleep. A lack of sleep is going to be enough to disrupt the hormones that are meant to regulate the appetite, the hormones of ghrelin, and leptin. Another hormone, known as cortisol, is going to get elevated any time that you are feeling stressed out.

Having these hormones fluctuate on a regular basis is going to increase your hunger and your cravings for foods that are not all that healthy, which is going to lead us to take in more calories in the process. In addition, studies have shown how a chronic level of sleep deprivation and chronic levels of stress especially when the two are combined, could be enough to increase your risk of several diseases, including obesity and type 2 diabetes.

Melanie Johnson

Chapter 13: Love Yourself

The majority of individuals don't think very much about self-improvement. We'd love to assist you to indulge in such a notion and find out just how much you can enjoy yourself. It's a requirement for accepting and creating your ideal weight and everything else that's fantastic for you. Just being conscious of the idea of self-help can move you farther along on the way of enjoying yourself and accepting yourself as you are. Your character and character are aware of the way you're feeling on your own. If you harbor bitterness or remorse, or sense undeserving, these emotions operate contrary to enjoying yourself.

- How can you see your flaws?

- Can you blame yourself? Self-love and finding an error or depriving yourself repaint each other. It is tough to enjoy yourself if you frequently find error ultimately.

- Can you put attention on negative aspects of yourself?

- Can you end up making self-deprecating statements, such as "I am not intelligent enough to..." or even "I am not great enough to..."?

- Can you punish yourself or refuse yourself?

- Can you establish boundaries with individuals who represent your very own moral and ethical criteria and your values and beliefs?

- Look at the mirror. How do you feel about yourself? Can you smile or frown?

- Which are you about the continuum of self?

- Are you currently respectful and admiring?

- Are you critical and judgmental, or would you love yourself for that you are?

- Have you been caring and caring this individual who you see?

If you're ambivalent, then contemplate these concerns further. Be truthful with yourself. Have a conversation on your own. Take a sincere look at yourself. Do not just examine your own body; examine your wisdom, your soul, your own emotions, along with your own heart. Know that: By enjoying yourself, you love yourself. If there's something that you can't accept on your own, be aware you could change that idea, and alter it to make anything you want, such as your ideal weight.

How Does It Feel to Love Yourself?

Have a look at these features. Are these familiar to you? It is the way it should feel if you like yourself:

- You genuinely feel happy and accepting your world, even though you might not agree with everything within it.

- You're compassionate with your flaws or less-than-perfect behaviours, understanding that you're capable of improving and changing.

- You mercifully love compliments and feel joyful inside.

- You frankly see your flaws and softly accept them learn to alter them.

- You accept all of the goodness that comes your way.

- You honour the great qualities and the fantastic qualities of everybody around you.

- You look at the mirror and smile (at least all the period).

Many confuse self-love with becoming arrogant and greedy. But some individuals are so caught up in themselves they make the tag of being egotistical and thinking just of these. We do not find that as a healthful self-indulgent, however, as a character which isn't well balanced in enjoying itself love and loving others.

It isn't selfish to get things your way; however, it's egotistical to insist that everybody else can see them your way too. The Dalai Lama states, "If you do not enjoy yourself, then you can't love other people. You won't have the capacity to appreciate others. If you don't have any empathy on your own, then you aren't capable of developing empathy for others" Dr. Karl Menninger, a psychologist, states it this way: "Self-love isn't opposed to this love of different men and women. You can't truly enjoy yourself and get yourself a favour with no people a favour, and vice versa." We're referring to the healthiest type of self-indulgent that simplifies the solution to accepting your best good.

Just take a better look at the way you see your flaws and blame yourself. Self-love and finding an error or depriving yourself isn't in any way compatible. If you deny enjoying yourself, you're in danger of paying too much focus on your flaws that is a sort of self-loathing.

You don't wish to place focus on negative aspects of yourself, for by keeping these ideas in your mind, you're giving them the psychological energy which brings that result or leaves it actual.

Self-love is positive energy. Blame, criticism, and faultfinding are energy. Self-hypnosis can help you utilize your mind-body to make new and much more loving ideas and beliefs on your own. It helps your mind-body create and take fluctuations in the patterns of feeling and thinking which have been for you for quite a while, and which aren't helpful for you. The trance work about the sound incorporates many positive suggestions to shift your ideas, emotions, and beliefs in alignment together with your ideal weight.

A Vital goal for all these positive hypnotic suggestions is the innermost feeling of enjoying yourself. If your self-loving feelings are constant with your ideal weight, then it is going to occur with increased ease. But if you harbour bitterness or remorse, or sense undeserving, these emotions operate contrary to enjoying yourself enough to think and take your ideal weight. Lucille Ball stated it well: "Love yourself first and everything falls in line" The hypnotic suggestions about the sound are directions for change led to the maximum "internal" degree of mind-body or unconscious. However, the "outer" changes in life action should also happen.

Many weight reduction methods you have been using might appear to be a lot of work. We suggest that by adopting a mindset that's without the psychological pressure related to "needing to," "bad or good," or even "simple or difficult," with no judgment in any way, the fluctuations could be joyous.

Yes, even joyous. It produces the whole journey of earning adjustments and shifting easier. The term "a labour of love" implies you enjoy doing this so much it isn't labour or responsibility. The "labour" of organizing a family feast in a vacation season, volunteering at a hospital or school, or even buying a gift for someone very particular can appear effortless. Here is the mindset that will assist you in following some weight loss methods. We invite you to place yourself in the situation of being adored.

You're doing so to you. Loving yourself eliminates the job, and that means it is possible to relish your advancement toward a lifestyle that encourages your ideal weight. Think about some action that you like to perform. Imagine yourself performing this action today. Notice that whenever you're doing something which you love to perform, you're feeling energized and beautiful, and some other attempt is evidenced by enjoyment. What is going on at these times is you see it absolutely "loving what you're doing." Sometimes, we recommend that you also find that as "enjoying yourself doing this." Maybe by directing more favourable attitude toward enjoying yourself, you'll end up enjoying what you're doing.

Lisa's Brimming Smile

After Lisa and Rick wed, both have been slender and appreciated active lifestyles which included softball and Pilates classes at the local gym. When their very first infant was first born, Lisa had obtained an additional fifteen lbs. From now, their infant came three decades later, and she had been twenty pounds' overweight. Depending on the demands of motherhood, she depended on fast-frozen foods, canned foods, and food to the table. Persistent sleep deprivation also maintained her power level reduced, and she can hardly keep up with the toddlers. Rick, a promising young company executive, took more and more duties on the job increasing the "ladder of success," indulging in company lunches, and even working late afternoon. He'd return home late; fall facing the TV and eat leftover pizza.

The youthful couple accepted their ancestral lifestyle but observed with dismay as their bodies grew tired and old beyond their years. However, they lasted. If their oldest boy entered astronomy, they became more upset. Small Ricky appeared to be the goal of each germfree, and he started to miss several days of college. If this was not enough, he also attracted the germs house to small brother, mother, and father. It appeared that four of these were with something that the whole winter.

The infant was colicky. From the spring, following a household bout with influenza, Lisa's friend supplied the title of a behavioural therapist who she explained could have the ability to shed some light about the recurrent diseases of Lisa's small boys. In the first consultation, Lisa declared the four decades of her household's lifestyle, culminating at current influenza where the small boys were recuperating. They were exhausted, tired, not sleeping well, and usually under sunlight. With summer vacation just around the corner, Lisa had been distressed to receive her family back on the right track.

The words of this nutritionist proved rather easy: Start feeding your household foods which are fresh and ready in your home. Start buying fruits and veggies, and make some simple recipes using rice and other grains. Learn how to create healthy and wholesome dishes to your loved ones. These phrases triggered Lisa to remember when she had been a kid about the time of her very own small boys. She remembered her mother fixing large fruit salads using lemon. She recalled delicious dishes of homemade soup along with hot fresh bread. At the instant, Lisa knew what she needed to make happen for her boys. And she'd make it occur. Approximately six months after, we received a telephone call from Lisa. I can hear the grin brimming in her voice. "You cannot think the shift in our loved ones. Ricky has had just one cold in the last six weeks, and we are all sleeping much better, and also the infant is happy and sleeping soundly during the night. Four days per week, we have a family walk after breakfast or after dinner. And guess what? I have lost thirty-five lbs., and that I was not dieting! I'm better than I have ever felt."

Giving Forth

Forgiveness is a significant step in enjoying yourself. At any time, you forgive, you're "committing forth" or "letting go" of a thing you're holding inside you. Let's be clear about this: bias is simply for you, not anybody else. It's not a kind of accepting, condoning, or justifying somebody else's activities. It's a practice of letting go of an adverse impression that has remained within you too long. It's the letting go of any emotion or idea which can be an obstacle between you and enjoying yourself and getting what you desire.

A lot of us are considerably more crucial and much tougher on ourselves than we're on the others. When you continue to notions of what you should or should not have completed, you're not enjoying yourself. Instead, you're putting alert energy to negative beliefs about yourself. Ideas like "I should have obtained a stroll" or even "I shouldn't have eaten this second slice of pie" can also be regarded as self-punishing. Sometimes, penalizing yourself, either by lack of overeating or eating, may even lead to discount for your wellbeing. By shifting your focus to self-appreciation, you go from the negative to the positive that is quite a bit more conducive to self-loving.

Melanie Johnson

Chapter 14: Portion Control

When you eat too quickly, you do not notice your stomach's cues that it is full. Eat slowly and listen to hunger cues to enhance feelings of fullness and ultimately, consume less food.

Improved Digestion

Many folks are there: That moment when you are through with Thanksgiving dinner and suddenly regret eating the maximum amount as you probably did. Once a year may not be that big of a deal; however, often consumption of large portions will cause a disturbance on your gastrointestinal system.

Considerably larger portion sizes contribute to an upset stomach and discomfort (caused by a distended stomach pushing down on your other organs). Your gastrointestinal system functions best when it is not full of food. Managing portions can help to get rid of cramping and bloating after eating. You furthermore may run the danger of getting pyrosis; as a result of having a full abdomen will push hydrochloric acid back into your digestive tract.

Money Savings

Eating smaller parts may lead to monetary benefits, mainly when eating out. In addition to eating controlled serving sizes, you do not have to purchase as many groceries. Measuring serving proportions can make the box of cereal and packet of nuts last longer than eating straight out of the container?

Adult portion sizes at restaurants will equal two, three, or even more servings. Therefore, immediately the food arrives at your table, request for a takeaway container and put away half of your food from the plate

How to Control Portions Using Hypnosis

Hypnosis can take you into a deeply relaxed state and quickly train your mind to understand when to do away with excess food instinctively, and allow your digestion to be lighter, and more comfortable. You may discover the pleasure of being in tune with what your own body requires nourishment. Hypnosis will re-educate your instincts to regulate hunger pangs. As you relax and repeatedly listen to powerful hypnotic suggestions that are going to be absorbed by your mind; you may quickly begin to note that:

- your mind is no longer engrossed in food
- your abdomen and gut feel lighter

- you now do not feel uncontrollable hunger pangs at 'non-meal' times

- you naturally forget to have food between meals

- you begin to enjoy a healthier lifestyle

There is a somewhat simple self-hypnosis process for helping you control your appetite and portions. In a shell, you are immersing yourself into a psychological state and picture a dial, or a flip switch of some type that is symbolic of your craving and your real hunger. Then you repeatedly apply to develop a true sense of control, and then you employ it out of the hypnotic state and when confronted with those things and circumstances to curb the perceived hunger and control your appetite.

Step 1: Get yourself into a comfortable position and one where you will remain undisturbed for the period of this exercise. Ascertain your feet are flat on the ground and hands not touching. Then once you are in position, calm yourself.

You can do that by using hypnosis tapes; they are basic processes to assist you in opening the door of your mind.

Step 2: You may prefer to deepen your hypnotic state. The best and most straightforward is imagining yourself in your favorite place and relaxing your body bit by bit. Keep focused on the session at hand (that is, watch out not to drift off) then go to the third step.

Step 3: Take a picture of a dial, a lever or a flippy switch of some kind that is on a box, or mounted on a wall of some sort- let it fully control your mind's eye. Notice the colors, the materials that it is created out of, and the way it indicates 0-10 to mark the variable degrees of your real hunger.

Notice wherever it is indicating currently- let it show you how hungry you are. Remember when last you ate, what you ate, whether or not the hunger is genuine or merely reacting to a recent bout of gluttony and wanting to gratify that sensation!

Once you have established the dial, where it is set, and trusting that the reading is correct, then go to the subsequent step.

Step 4: Flip the dial down a peg and notice the effects taking place within you. Study your feedback and ascertain that it feels like you are moving your appetite with the dial. The more you believe you are affecting your appetite with the dial, the more practical its application in those real-life situations.

Practice turning it down even lower and start recognizing how you use your mind to change your perceived appetite utilizing a method that is healthy and helps keep you alert when you encounter circumstances with plenty of food supply. Tell yourself that the more you observe this, the better control you gain over your appetite.

You might even create a strong affirmation that accompanies this dial "I am in control of my eating" is one such straightforward statement. Word it as you wish and make sure it is one thing that resonates well with you. Once you have repeated the meaningful affirmations to yourself severally with conviction, proceed to the next step.

Step 5: Visualize yourself during a future scenario, where there is going to be constant temptation to continue eating although you are full, or to consume an excessive amount. See the sights of that place, take a mental note of the other people there, notice the smells, and hear the sounds. Become increasingly aware of how you are feeling in this place. Get the most definition and clarity possible then notice that once the temptation presents itself, you turn down the dial on your craving. You realize that you are not hungry to eat anymore, then repeat your positive affirmations to yourself a few more times to strengthen it.

Run through this future state of affairs severally on loop to make sure your mind is mentally rehearsed about your plan to respond.

Step 6: Twitch your little finger and toes, then open your eyes and proceed to observe your skills in real-life and spot how much control you have.

Practice the hypnosis for many days before going to face temptation, just to make sure that the process is firmly lodged into your mind. Unless hypnosis has positively compelled you or somebody close to you to shop for a new, smaller wardrobe, it is going to be arduous to believe that this "mind-over-body" approach may assist you to get a handle on food consumption.

Seeing is Believing Concepts

So, see for yourself. You ought not to be delighted by a number of tall tales of weight-loss using hypnosis. The following concepts contain several suggestions for altering your diet, appetite, and serving portions.

Your Solution Lies Within

Hypnotherapists believe that everything you would likely need to succeed is within your reach. You do not want the newest drug or another absurd diet. Slimming is about trusting your innate talents, as you do while driving a car. You will forget how terrified you were for your first driving lesson. However, you maintained the lessons until you could drive without much thought or effort. Similarly, losing weight could appear beyond your reach; however, it is merely a matter of striking your balance.

What You Think You Can Achieve

This applies to hypnosis as well as real life. Subjects who expect results often receive them. The expectation of being helped is essential. You should think and expect your hypnosis weight loss strategy to work.

Intensify the Positive

Aversive or negative thoughts will work for a moment; however, if you hope for lasting transformation, you will want to assume a more positive demeanor. There is an exciting example of one 50-year-old woman who lost more than fifty pounds. She repeats daily: "Unnecessary food could be a burden on my body. I intend to shed what I do not need."

If You Visualize It, It Will Come

Visualizing success prepares you for a victorious reality, much like athletes do. At the beginning of each day, images of clean, healthy eating help you imagine the required steps to turning into that healthy eater. Is imagination too burdening a task? If so, find a photograph of when you were at your most comfortable weight and start there. Try to remember your routines and find out what you can do differently at the present moment. Or perhaps visualize obtaining a recommendation from a future older, wiser self when she has necessarily attained her desired weight.

Send Away Food Cravings

Hypnotherapists habitually harness the ability of symbolic representation. Invite your mind to place food cravings on a white cloud or in a helium balloon and send them floating up, up, up, and away.

Invest in More Than One Strategy

When it comes to shedding weight and keeping it off, a winning duo is cognitive-behavioral therapy (CBT) and hypnosis that helps work out harmful thoughts and behaviors. Raising awareness each smart hypnotherapist is aware of, could be a crucial step toward lasting change. Before attempting hypnotherapy, keep a record of everything you ingest for a week or two.

Modify as Often as Necessary

Melanie Johnson

The importance of applying existing patterns has been emphasized repeatedly. Instead of submitting to a craving of a pint of ice cream, you can modify the calories craving to perhaps a cup of frozen Greek yogurt.

Melanie Johnson

Chapter 15: Perfect Mind, Perfect Weight

Perfect thoughts and ideal weight. The term may seem like a fantasy to you. What are the archetypal mind and ideal weight? They're the realistic conditions you'll be able to use as you pursue fat reduction. "Realistic?" You inquire. "How can anything be 'ideal,' let alone my burden and my ideas about my burden?" Well, recall what we said about the strength of believing and belief. Can it serve your curiosity to desire or hope to anything less than perfection on your own? Indulge us for some time as we clarify why you're able to think your mind and burden because "perfect."

Perfect fat is your weight that's ideal for you. It's the weight that's attainable and consistent with everything you need and precisely what you're ready to give yourself and accept. More to the point, your ideal weight provides you with a healthy body, the human body which goes effortlessly, and also the one where you are feeling great about yourself and joyful. And what are ideal thoughts? You presently have a mind. It's flawless. But there can be a few ideas in those ideal thoughts of yours that are providing you with undesirable outcomes. There can be something that you remember, possibly habits or routines, which provide you with undesirable outcomes. However, you may use your ideal head to match your ideas to offer you precisely what you desire. It's possible to use your head to accomplish the bodyweight that you desire.

IN THE TWINKLING OF AN EYE,

Your current body is the consequence of your ideas and beliefs. You've chosen these ideas and beliefs by the way you live, which generated your current weight. You haven't made any errors, regardless of what you may be thinking of yourself. Instead, you've just experienced undesirable outcomes. These undesirable effects are an immediate effect of misaligned ideas and beliefs about you, which are the patterns of behavior or way of life. The Quick weight loss diet is all about using your perfect thoughts to match with your ideas to provide you with the results you desire. You honestly can use your head to accomplish the bodyweight you desire. Let's examine a few of the learning which has occurred in your life that will let you know where you're now together with your body weight. Can you wake up one afternoon, and feel additional pounds? Or could it be a slow accumulation with time? Or perhaps you've understood nothing else as early youth. Whatever the situation, there are lots of factors that made your body:

- Food options
- Eating customs
- That the self-critic in you
- Economic history
- Psychological history
- Impact of household
- Impact of buddies
- Cultural heritage

These and some other variables were discovered in your lifetime and became the beliefs, which subsequently became routines of activity that generated your body. We'll be more unique. Notice that these aspects appear authentic for you in your last years. In other words, consider what you did understand about your youth about eating and food.

- What kinds of grocery stores did your household buy?

- What foods do your parents cook, and were they typically ready?

- Do you eat only at home or often grab food?

- Have you been served fresh, healthy, high-calorie foods, or do you eat mainly processed and extremely processed foods, fried foods, and "junk" foods?

- Were you aware or focus on nutrition, or has there been any irresponsible disregard for what your household ate?

- What did you find out about eating mindfully?

- Were you educated that healthful food options led to healthy bodies?

- Did anybody teach you how you can understand what's healthy food and what's not?

- Is your meal selections based on what is tasted or seemed high or priceless?

- Can your loved ones or college instruct you about healthy bodies and audio nourishment, or has it been the "nutrition education" through TV advertisements and food makers' advertising?

What exactly did you learn as a kid? What're your beliefs about eating food, along with your entire body? Analyze your own socioeconomic or socio-cultural roots and see whether they had an effect on the way and what you've learned to consume. Over thirty-five years back, sociological research pointed out weight issues in the working and lower class according to their intake patterns of what's been known as "poverty-level foods." Like hot dogs, canned meats, and processed luncheon meats. Cultural groups also have been analyzed to understand their nutritional patterns and meals, like eating with lard or ingesting a diet of fried and high-fat foods, which can lead to higher body fat loss. These influences can readily be accepted because they're "regular" into the category, of course. Then let's take a look in the teen years. During adolescence, Are there some changes in your weight loss? Just as a boy, have you been invited to pile more food on your plate? "Look at him, consume! Certainly, he will develop to a large guy!" (There's a telling metaphor) Or are you currently admonished to eat? When you're a budding young woman, did a smart girl take you under her wing and then the marvel of menses and the wonderment of body modifications.

Such as the organic growth in body fat with all the evolution of breasts and broader hips? Were you conscious during puberty, that unless your body improved body fat by 22 percent, it wouldn't correctly grow and create menses? Or was that "hushed up" within an awkward improvement? It was likely during adolescence that you heard there's a stigma in obese men and women. Spend a couple of minutes writing down the aspects that appear to be accurate for you in your last years. Ponder the encounters and influences which are forming your body. In high school, the athletes at college sports have always been a healthful weight and are the cheerleaders and homecoming queens.

Melanie Johnson

What ancient beliefs regarding your popularity and self-image could have formed from your social interactions in high school? What did you understand about physical activity, and what customs did you produce? Have you been introduced to physical activity as part of a healthful way of life, through family or sports outings of walks or hikes? Or was that the blaring TV a regular fixture, enticing everybody to the sofa? Next is a matter which most people have never been aware of throughout their development. As you're growing up, have you sought the attention of self-care based on trendy clothes, makeup, and hairstyles, or about healthful food, routine physical activity, along with spiritual and intellectual nourishment? What about today? Spend a couple more minutes writing down the aspects that appear to be accurate for you in the past couple of decades. What influences and experiences formed the ideas, which turned in the beliefs that turned into your body?

After high school, you moved away from the house. Suddenly you no longer agree with your family's life. Are you aware of your options or can you start eating with blow off? If you in a close connection, just what compromises or arrangements about foods and physical activity did you input into too? Most associations develop from similar pursuits, including food preferences and eating styles. In the end, the relationship comprises eating routines and tastes, which are a consequence of compromise. Have your connections encouraged smart food choices and healthy eating? Maybe you've experienced pregnancy. Can you learn the way to get a wholesome pregnancy and then nourish a healthy infant within you? Or did you put in pounds after giving birth? How did your lifestyle assist you in recovering your typical fat or suppressing it? If you were active in the league or sports games, did your livelihood or family duties take priority and eliminate these physical fitness tasks from your regular basics? Can you correct exercise and diet too, or even did the fat begin to collect? Did an accident, injury, or disease happen that disrupted a reasonable physical action that has been supportive of healthy fat?

Because you can see, the way you got to where you're now was no crash. You heard from the folks about you, or you also consumed out of the surroundings --the best way to create food decisions, the way to eat, and the way to look after yourself emotionally and physically. Whether the thoughts you heard were tremendous and healthy or not so high and not as healthy, they became your own beliefs, and eventually became you and your own body. Bear in mind that you didn't do anything wrong. However, you need to experience the outcomes of eating and living, which have been consistent with your ideas and beliefs.

Through time, what has been your answer to individuals and their opinions about your weight loss, bad or good? Can you go out and purchase a fantastic pair of sneakers, or do you consume to facilitate psychological distress? Maybe you even heard the latter response on your youth. Did your mom ever provide you with a plateful of food to comfort you when you're miserable? These are learned answers, and they may be unlearned and replaced with new answers and routines to make your ideal weight. Just ask, "Just how long does this happen?" We inform you, "In the twinkling of the eye," For the minute that you understand that you need it sufficient to get anything to possess it, it's completed. You've just altered the management of highly efficient energy in you, which will be directed at figuring out how to attain the outcome which you need, your ideal weight.

Your Perfect Mind Relearning

It's simple to comprehend how you got or "heard" to contemplate over your ideal weight. And it'll be simple to create new decisions, to relearn new routines, and also to make new and much more healthful habits. How can we learn? We know by mimicking another Individual, analyzing books (such as this one), with other tools, and practicing the activities which make the outcomes we seek. The best and lasting learning entails repetition and practice. It is essential to practice in the best possible way.

Pretend to be a violinist for a minute, and you're searching for a grand symphony operation in New York City. There are two ways in which you practice. The first that is entirely ineffective would be to play with that tough segment fast, over and over and above, always playing precisely the very same mistakes—but trusting that your palms will play it properly.

The critical thing is that you're giving your focus on practicing correctly. By being aware of what you're practicing, and also the way you're practicing it, you're studying the new routines which are replacing the last routines. You're practicing the action that generates your ideal body weight. You, too, can make "muscle" by practicing mindful eating (eating slowly, chewing thoroughly, swallowing the last bite until you take another bite) or even a more cautious, slower fork-to-mouth motion. You can also exercise a whole dining style, which becomes conditioned as mind-body learning or memory, which instantly becomes automatic. As it becomes an automatic or second character, you don't need to think about doing it.

Melanie Johnson

Melanie Johnson

Chapter 16: Daily Weight Loss Motivation with Mini Habits

Stress and Emotions

My guess is that one of the challenges you have faced is stress and emotional eating? You are not alone. According to the American Psychological Association (APA), 43 percent of women surveyed said they ate in response to stress in the last month. Many women said that eating in response to stress didn't make them feel better, only more guilty and bad about themselves and their bodies. So, even though the rational mind knows a bagel isn't going to solve the fact that a boyfriend didn't send a Valentine card or that the chocolate cookie isn't a cure for having to sit down and do taxes, the Weight Struggler eats when she's upset anyway.

Emotion, Stress, and The Brain

Our mind and body evolved to move from 0 to 100 milliseconds to get us out of danger as fast as possible. This fight-or-flight response enhanced survival back in the day. When fear or danger happens today, the same fantastic survival mechanism occurs. The hormone cortisol floods the system, and the reptilian brain literally shuts down the conscious, rational-thinking brain. It says "Hey, there's no time to think—JUST MOVE THOSE FEET!" Almost instantly, every bit of energy goes to preparing us to flee as fast as possible.

The problem is that the reptilian brain does not know how to differentiate between a lion and bumper-to-bumper traffic, the yelling boss, or a bad hair day. The mind interprets any change in "normal" as a threat, triggering release of cortisol to prep the body for a lightning-fast getaway. Stress also shifts the brain into a reward-seeking state, because it associates the reward state to "feeling better."

Eating may be a calming reward, but eventually it also makes the Weight Struggler feel bad. Only 16 percent of women in the APA survey reported that the food they turned to for comfort actually helped.

Cinder-struggler

In the summer before my senior year, I quit my part-time mushroom job and joined Weight Watchers. I had never been so heavy in all my life. I felt ashamed as I got on the scale in front of the nice lady who reminded me of my grandmother and she called out my weight. "192 pounds!" It was a humiliating moment. Had it really come to this?

I was only 16, but I felt like I was 100 years old. My body ached and I didn't move well. I didn't fit into any cute clothes like those my friends wore, and I had never been out on a real date. I hung out with guys, but no one looked at me as girlfriend material. I was just the funny fat friend.

I needed to do something. I thought I couldn't go into my senior year looking and feeling like this. My struggle was consuming every waking minute of my day. So, I embraced the Weight Watchers plan and stuck to it. I had to make it work, and I found I had enough willpower to "be good" on the plan week after week.

Melanie Johnson

I was losing weight and feeling excited about my progress. I cherished my weight loss card that showed each week's weight victory. I was in control, and as long as I was "good," I would keep getting my weight loss payoff. There were other payoffs too. I could wear normal-sized clothes. People seemed to treat me with more respect, too.

The dark side of this rather magical time of being a star Weight Watcher was that I still felt like a Weight Struggler on the inside. Would I be able to keep this charade up forever? I pushed the dark thoughts aside and just kept going with the program.

Cinder-Struggler Goes to the Ball

I hit my weight goal of 134 pounds in Weight Watchers in the spring of 1982. I remember being called up in front of my weekly meeting for my goal weight award and feeling so proud, emotional, and like I had arrived. This fantastic feeling lasted less than 24 hours.

The very next day I was sitting in the lunchroom, selling tickets for the senior breakfast with the other girls on the committee when I was asked to the prom, in front of the entire lunchroom, by the captain of the swim team. We were in the spring musical together, but I didn't know him well. I sat there dumbfounded, mouth gaping, as the lunchroom fell silent and waited for my response. "Yes," I said rather meekly but loud enough to cause a roar among those listening. I felt dizzy. Was this really happening?

Now you would think after two stunning wins like hitting your goal weight and being asked to the senior prom by one of the most popular guys in school would have you feeling on the top of the world, and I did...for a moment.

I walked home from school on cloud nine, my heart racing. My emotions were soaring so high that I couldn't take them all in. When I got home, I went immediately to the kitchen and without even thinking began to eat everything. I pulled crackers and peanut butter out of the cupboard along with chocolate chip cookies and milk from the fridge. It seemed like I had a bottomless hole to fill. I tried to stop it, but any conscious-mind protests were run right over by my subconscious mind's need to eat my way back to calmness and an emotional status quo.

Over the next few weeks before the prom, my emotions were all over the place, and so was my eating. I tried to get back to that magical spot on the Weight Watchers plan where I was before the prom invitation. I could be suitable for a few days, but then the dam would break, and I would binge away all the unfamiliar feelings. I was like a gazelle running from the lion of emotions swirling inside me.

I made my prom dress from a cool Vogue pattern four weeks before the prom. On the night of the prom, I discovered I couldn't zip the dress all the way. I had tried it on the last week and it fit. It was snug but it worked. Now that zipper wouldn't close! I panicked and began to cry.

Melanie Johnson

My wonderful mother thought fast on her feet and never once brought up what we both knew—I had gained weight. The stress-eating had driven me out of my prom dress. Mom handed me a jacket that went pretty well with the dress and covered both the partly unzipped back of my dress and my humiliation.

Anyone who saw me that night at the prom would have seen a girl dancing and having fun. Inside, though, my heart was broken. I had proven yet again that my Weight Struggler beliefs were true. I was a failure. My bad habits hadn't gone away; they were just temporarily dormant. Now they were back with a vengeance. There I was like Cinderella. The clock hadn't struck midnight, but I was already turning back into a weight-struggling pumpkin.

Meditation for Mindful Eating

This meditation is going to be focused on eating mindfully. You might even try this one (after you have already completed it once) while you are eating as a new method. Listen to this directly or repeat the script in your own voice and use that to help guide you through the meditation. Find a comfortable position and begin when you are ready. Let these thoughts flow through your mind naturally as if you were saying them.

I can feel each breath that enters and exits my body. I am very aware of my breath. I am able to tell how much air is entering my body, and how much air is leaving as well. I am focused on nothing but the breath that is coming in and out of my mouth. As I become relaxed, I am imagining myself eating.

I am sitting behind a plate filled with delicious foods that will keep me full. I know that the best way to keep me interested in my meal is to include various parts and food groups.

Having whole grains will keep me full longer. Veggies will give me fiber and fruits give me that sweetness I need. All of these foods keep me happy not just while I am eating them, but throughout the day.

They are not just good for my body, but for my mind as well.

I feel each bite as it enters my mouth. I love the blend of the textures as I chew into each bite.

My teeth are healthy and powerful enough to be able to tear up anything from the meat of an animal to the hardest of apples. I am powerful as I chew into my food, feeling the textures in my mouth. It feels good to replenish my body. I enjoy the sustenance I get from these delicious meals.

I don't need to eat large bites. Small bites are just as effective. I used to eat more massive spoonful's, filling my mouth as much as I could. Now I know that it's better to take smaller bites so I can focus instead on the flavor and not just the amount of food that I'm eating. I'm concerned with texture and taste, not just eating more to keep me full.

The slower I chew my food, the less I have to digest with my body. This will make it easier to pull the nutrients from my food.

I can feel this gave me energy. I am absorbing as much as I can from this food. I am taking all the nutrients and minerals that it has to offer. All of the components of my food will help me to be a more reliable and healthier person.

I know that as I let food enter my mouth, I am putting right nutrients inside my body. As I eat slowly, I realize that I don't even need to eat seconds. I can be delighted with the first amount that I chose to eat.

I take smaller portions so that if I do want seconds, I am not eating that much. I also like to use smaller plates now because I know that the food seems more significant to me. There are so many things that I can do to help me focus my attention on mindful eating rather than the mindless practices I used to do while consuming my food.

I am relaxed as I eat, not forcing myself to chew too fast. There is no rush. When I am feeling rushed to eat,

Melanie Johnson

I make sure only to eat a snack. I am eating my food in
a relaxed state.

Melanie Johnson

Chapter 17: Shed Tummy Fat Using the Exercise Strategy

Exercise is as crucial as correct nutrition, and without use, it is virtually impossible to get to a single percentage of body fat. Your exercise program has to consist of both cardio and weight training. Working out three times a week is good enough if you have not done much physical exercise before. The less body fat you have, the more you have to work to eliminate it.

Make it your lifestyle to live healthy if you want to live a healthy life. You can start by exercising regularly. You can go to the gym and spend at least two hours of lifting weights every week. Or, if you don't have time to work out, always incorporate physical activities in your routine. Instead of taking the elevator, you can take the stairs when transferring from one floor to the other.

If you're current routine is the same old weight lifting and some cardio, then that is going to have to change today,

Problem one: The reason is, your body isn't being pushed and kicked into fat loss overdrive. This is where your present exercise strategy comes to be an issue; this is because our collection can be familiar with specific uniformities, as an example, your routine Monday through Friday routine is now a regular regimen that your body has adapted to.

So what are you going to do to give your body a little shock? It's called high-intensity interval training. This kind of workout is how you can start boosting your metabolic process and start burning fat.

Melanie Johnson

The workout is composed of any type of activity such as weight training, staircase climbing, cycling, and also or any kind of cardio of your choice. After your extending and workouts, you will start your workout nonstop at full maximum for 30 to 60 secs. This is where you will go full speed and 100%. You will take a remainder period of either 30-60 secs after that and repeat the process six to eight times.

This exercise below will press your fat loss metabolism in very high equipment; the intensity level is so high that your body is compelled to start burning that fat and make you leaner. You can do a mixture of different exercises as long as your rest periods are regular.

If you are to integrate this training program with a healthy diet plan, your belly fat will start disappearing before you know it. It functions, understandable and straightforward, but you need to show consistency for some weeks. You'll wind up giving your body no choice but to start shedding the fat.

The problem with most people is that it is easier to gain weight than to shed it. When we have been a bit careless about our diet for long, eventually we need to start thinking of the best way to minimize abdominal fat, because the fat is located where its challenging to eliminate for the majority of people. You need to be stubborn because the fat can be persistent.

Eating much less healthy meals as well as being careless is far also very easy. Envision if you just took the possibility every day to make all the simple points to obtain exercise. Taking the stairs instead of the elevator and walking your kids to school as opposed to taking the family car.

Melanie Johnson

Some of us have jobs where we take a seat every working hours of the day and also get little or no possibility to stand and relocate. All these factors result in one crucial point - fat storage.

Overweight is not in charge of your physique; you will need to make a change and take action if you feel stressed out. However, personally, how do you do it when you don't have time to exercise? After returning from work and putting the kids to rest, it's too late in the night, and you may be too exhausted to exercise. The adhering to tip is what you can do during the day, at your work or anywhere, to gradually start shedding tummy fat.

Cardiovascular Exercises

One more point that you can enter into to discover how to shed stubborn belly fat quick for men is to do cardio exercises and include it in your exercise regimens. These cardio workouts might consist of cycling, running, trekking, swimming, roller skating, and quick walking.

Abdominal exercises

How to burn stomach fat quickly for men may have something to do with the various kinds of abdominal workouts. This is why you must discover how to integrate these exercises right into your routine.

Right here are some workouts that may be helpful to you:

Melanie Johnson

Abdominal muscle Twist - Should be done with fifteen reps on each side.

--Bike Crunch- ought to be done by alternating the activities of the arm joints with the knees.

--Oblique Crunch- need to be done together with breathing exercises in fifteen repeatings during the regimen.

These are some of the most detailed techniques that you require to find out for you to recognize how to burn stubborn belly fats fast for men. By just complying with these pointers, you will be able to melt those fats precisely and securely. Naturally, in addition to a healthy diet, you will have the ability to keep the fitness and health of your body.

Work on Your Muscles

There's a strategy that everyone can do many times a day before you eat. For effective results, you ought to do it after you have eaten as well. What to do?

Leg crouches with your body as the only weight!

Do squats for 60 - 90 secs right before each dish and do as much after you have eaten.

Why?

Because it brings blood sugar level carrier (GLUT-4) to the surface of muscle mass cells, meaning opening up more gateways for the power to flow right inside.

This is helping you, considered that the more gateways we've obtained open before insulin turns on the same

GLUT-4 on the fat cells, the more we can put in muscles in contrast to fat!

If you want to go all-in trying to bring a more GLUT-4 to your muscular tissue cells, you can include a tricep exercise to the "exercise." Prolong your arms against a wall surface and do a push-up activity towards the wall. This will engage your arm muscle mass as much as called for.

It might look difficult to do these kinds of exercises both before and after every meal. My tip to you is to do the triceps and squats workouts inside the toilet or any other area where you can keep to yourself.

I'm sure you've been through this situation, if not directly, you know someone who has: they've made use of the most recent diet program that assured them weight management in three days together with a permanent weight reduction to comply with, only to backfire: the fat returned, which with a vengeance.

Well, the reality is a long-term weight reduction needs something more excellent than adhering to the latest trend diet program. It requires a full change in understanding, life, action, and diet style. But you do not need to fret: this can be attained gradually.

So if you are after a long-term weight reduction, you need to comply with these few easy steps:

1. Minimize fats in your day-to-day food. Lowering fats will help your goal because high-fat diets have extra calories than routine food, in some cases, the ratio is as much as 2:1

2. Start eating more vegetables and fruits.

This is easy. With each lunch, ensure you have a good plate of fresh vegetables with it: one cut cucumber, a tomato, an excellent eco-friendly fleshy pepper, maybe a half-peeled carrot. Pour a healthy salad dressing on it to enhance the taste if you like. When you are starving, start munching on an apple, or a banana, or a pear.

3. Before going to the grocery, eat.

Have a sandwich, a healthy snack, and even a routine dish. Whatever you do, don't go shopping on an empty belly. You often tend to get stay off some things when you're hungry, and many stuff' will inevitably include a lot of points that are not healthy and balanced for you, a whole lot of junk food, sugary foods, and alcohol.

You are using the swimming pool. Swimming is not just the best for weight-loss, but it strengthens the muscles of your entire body will bring out your abs.

4. Shift your thinking.

You need to start thinking 'health' instead of 'diet.' When we think of diet, we associate it with pain, with struggle, with a difficult choice of foods to go through.

Health means looking younger, better, and enjoying life more. Once you have a healthy attitude, everything will come along nicely.

Start with any of these tips, not necessarily in order, and not even necessary to do them all now. Start small, but start somewhere and don't give up. Start with little thing, and once your brain and your body get used to the change and accept it, you will know. And then, take the next small change. Before you know it, you have embarked on a permanent weight loss journey, which is here to stay permanently.

If you are to combine this training program with a solid diet plan, your belly fat will start disappearing before your eyes. You'll end up giving your body no choice but to start burning the fat away.

When we have been a bit careless about our diet for too long, at some point, we have to start thinking about the best way to reduce abdominal fat. The following tip is what you can do during the day, at your work or anywhere else, to start shedding belly fat gradually.

Reducing fats will help with your goal because high-fat foods have more calories than regular food, sometimes the ratio is as much as 2:1

Melanie Johnson

Chapter 18: Optimal Nutrition

Eating Healthy Vs. Achieving Your Goal Physique

With the idea of attaining a fantastic body, folks instantly consider eating healthy. Nevertheless, eating healthful foods does not automatically mean that you're achieving your target body. While obtaining your very best body does not exactly mean that you're eating healthy. To eat healthily means typically you give your body with sufficient nutrients to operate effectively. Your body needs a particular number of micronutrients (vitamins and minerals) and macronutrients (carbohydrates, proteins, and carbohydrates) so as to operate in its very best ability. It's your duty to satisfy your body's nutrient requirements so as to keep decent health. Reaching a fantastic body usually involves losing weight or gaining muscle. To be able to lose excess weight, a person must maintain a calorie deficit wherever your body burns off more calories than the number of calories you eat and drink. Gaining weight requires you to do the contrary, at which in a calorie excess you have more calories than the amount the body burns off calories off.

Though eating healthful foods has unlimited benefits, It's just as essential to satisfy the necessity of attaining your exercise goal. By way of example, if your objective is to burn fat and you also eat 10,000 calories worth of veggies every day, you are eating healthy but are consuming a lot of calories to achieve your objective.

Because of this, it's best to consume towards your target body when keeping excellent health.

What's a Calorie?

You hear about calories all of the time, but what does it mean? A calorie is a device that measures energy. The food that you eat is not measured in size or weight, but by how much energy it's. If you hear something that includes 100 calories, it is a method of describing just how much energy that your body might gain from drinking or eating it. As the quantity of gas pumped into a vehicle is measured in gallons, different food, or beverages you eat is measured in calories. The body breaks down food in an exceptional manner, so the number of calories is a means of understanding how much energy your system will get from whatever you eat or drink. 'Calorie' is only a specific phrase for 'energy'.

Are Calories Bad For You?

Calories aren't bad for you because the body needs them to get energy. Nevertheless, eating a lot of calories and not burning off enough of these off through physical activity may cause weight gain with time. Consuming too small calories over time won't enable your body to work correctly and may have a negative impact on your wellbeing. Foods like lettuce contain hardly any calories (1 cup of shredded lettuce has less than 10 calories), whereas foods such as peanuts have a great deal of calories (1/2 cup of peanuts contains

427 calories daily). Understanding how many calories your body requires each day can allow you to select which foods are right for you.

How Does Your Body Use Calories?

Your body requires calories simply to remain alive and function properly. This energy is utilized for essential functions like maintaining your heart beating and lung breathing. Calories are crucial for several fundamental and intricate functions such as the regulation of body temperature as well as also the functioning of each cell in the human entire body. The more activity you do will be that the more calories you burn off. Your body also requires calories so as to grow and grow. You burn calories before considering it as during the digestion of food, recovery of muscles after exercise, as well as while you are sleeping.

How Many Calories Do You Want?

Folks differ in size and have different metabolisms; therefore, the quantity of calories an individual should eat will change based upon many things. These factors include an individual's height, age, weight, and daily activity level. The larger an individual is, the more calories a person could want, vice versa. Although two individuals can have exactly the identical body dimensions, the number of calories that they want can differ due to the way their body adjusts exactly what they eat. Calorie calculators are available on the internet, which may be employed to ascertain the number of calories your body requires dependent on the vital facets. If you consume many calories than your body wants, then the additional calories are converted to fat. If you consume fewer calories then you require, then your system uses your stored body fat as the energy it needs to function. Knowing the number of calories you want can allow you to control your weight.

Macro Basics

Macronutrients or macros are carbs, fats, and protein. Together with the expression "macro," meaning quite big, these three nutrients are responsible for supplying calories (the only other material that supplies calories is alcohol however isn't a macronutrient because we don't want it for survival). Whatever that you eat is broken down into those three macronutrients. Your body doesn't recognize the food that you consume as "poultry, sausage, rice, etc.". Rather, your entire body sees anything you eat as a carbohydrate, fat, or protein. This is why you find these macronutrients written in bold letters to the nutrition label of any food or beverage product.

What's a Carb?

Carbohydrate is the body's main source of energy. There are 2 kinds of carbohydrates, complex and simple. A very simple carbohydrate supplies your body with rapid energy but does not last long. An intricate carbohydrate takes more time to break down on your body, nevertheless it is a long-lasting supply of energy.

Melanie Johnson

Neither simple nor complex carbohydrate is bad for you. They could both be utilized to your benefit throughout the day. Upon waking in the morning, you likely have not had anything to eat for the past couple of hours you have been asleep. Therefore it is sometimes a fantastic idea to eat simple carbohydrates for instant energy. If you intend on being from home for a couple of hours, complex carbohydrates are a great selection for its long-term steady energy. So integrating both kinds of carbohydrates in your diet may permit you better to manage your levels of energy throughout the day.

Examples of complex carbohydrates include whole grains like whole Wheat bread, oatmeal, and brown rice alongside other foods like sweet potato and beans. Simple carbs include foods like fruits, white bread, white rice, white potatoes, veggies, juice, pop tarts, etc.

Melanie Johnson

Sugar is a simple carbohydrate that comes in various forms like sugar, fructose, lactose, sucrose, etc. Though both simple and intricate carbohydrates are broken down to glucose within the body, absorption and digestion are the principal differences between both different types.

What Is Protein?

Protein helps build and repair tissue when playing a role in various cell functions within the body. It's a significant element for growing nails, hair, muscle, and different areas of the human body. Amino acids are building blocks of protein. An entire protein includes all 20 amino acids, even while the lack of one or more amino acids is known as an incomplete protein.

Melanie Johnson

Complete proteins are primarily found in meats like poultry, beef, beef, fish in addition to legumes, milk, and whey protein. Foods like grains, seeds, nuts, or beans are considered incomplete proteins. It's encouraged to eat at least 0.8 - 1.2 g of protein per 1 pound of your body weight for optimum muscle development. With several unique forms of protein in the marketplace which range from the origin, absorption rate, and procedure of filtration, any comprehensive protein is helpful for the growth and repair of muscle. Poultry, fish, milk, legume, soy, whey, and other resources of proteins have their differences, but any comprehensive protein is of fantastic advantage for repairing and building muscle. The crucial thing is to find sufficient protein to satisfy your body's need for optimum growth.

What Is Fat?

Fat controls hormones, aides from the transportation of cells, and makes it feasible for different nutrients to finish tasks within the body. Fat can also be your body's secondary source of vitality. When your body doesn't have sufficient carbohydrates easily available, it uses fat as an alternative source of gas. As a result, the notion of burning fat is to limit the quantity of primary energy (carbohydrates) so the body is able to utilize its secondary resource of energy (body fat). Various kinds of fats contain saturated fat, polyunsaturated, monounsaturated, and trans-fat. It's encouraged to steer clear of trans-fat because of its health advantages. While every kind of fat has its own advantages and disadvantages, it's helpful to look closely at the whole amount of fat in a single product.

Foods that have a high number of fats include peanut butter, oils, avocado, and nuts. Consuming low levels of fat over the years may lead to hormone levels to become erratic, which makes it important to have enough even while attempting to burn off fat. The quantity of fat required daily could vary anywhere from 15 percent to over 40 percent of total calories based on the person and fitness target.

Quality of Weight Loss or Weight Gain

If you're in a calorie deficit where your body burns off more calories than you eat, then you are going to eliminate weight. This doesn't automatically make sure that the entire weight you lose is only going to come from fat. Your body is composed of lean mass, fat, and fat. This implies any weight that's lost or obtained may come from any one of those three. When shedding fat, you risk losing weight, and if gaining weight, you risk placing on excess fat. Not monitoring macros puts you at a higher risk for muscle loss and fat gain since you would not understand how many calories you're becoming. Consuming the ideal amount of protein, fat, and carbohydrates helps to make sure you keep muscle while shedding weight, and restrict the rise of body fat while incorporating muscle.

More Energy, Better Mood

Melanie Johnson

Carbohydrates are the body's most important source of energy, therefore getting too little carbohydrates over time may leave you feeling exhausted and contribute to inadequate workout functionality. By properly setting up your macros, you optimize the number of carbohydrates you can consume while burning off fat. If you may eat more food while losing weight, then why not make the most of Fat is in charge of controlling your own hormones, therefore not having sufficient can lead to an imbalance that could result in mood swings and other undesirable symptoms. It's normal to drop short of your everyday fat requirements by merely eating "clean" foods that typically include little to no fat. Consuming low fat and carbohydrates over time may allow you to feel exceptionally miserable. To believe losing weight is a struggle, why make it tougher on yourself to accomplish your objective.

Melanie Johnson

Chapter 19: Healthy Habits are Necessary

The limbic framework is an old piece of our cerebrum that contains various programmed forms worried about endurance, including our enthusiastic responses. Feelings regularly work as delivery people that furnish us with relevant data. Envision that a feeling resembles a conveyance individual who has a significant bundle to get to you, and he won't stop until it's conveyed. A large number of our feelings are intended to be awkward because they should persuade us to accomplish something, for example, move away from danger. Shockingly, our cutting-edge world frequently presents us with saw dangers that we can't escape from; there's nothing we can "do," however, we despite everything get the passionate responses. For instance, have you at any point been irate while sitting in rush hour gridlock? Or on the other hand, stressed over what the future may bring? Congrats! You're a well-working individual.

A treat or a beverage of liquor or smoke to manage a distressing day or an awful state of mind, at that point you realize that feelings can assume a significant job in our capacity to adhere to our healthy habits. Feeling travelers regularly thump us off our course. We will investigate our feeling travelers and create aptitudes to manage them, so we're better ready to adhere to our habits course.

Melanie Johnson

Our Fix-It Brain

Recall our great critical thinking mind? It has been a helpful device for people in our development. Shockingly it gets a kick out of the chance to take a shot at fixing—or disposing of our sentiments, which can push us into difficulty. Take, for instance, my customer Anna. She came to me since she believed she was drinking excessively. We immediately found that she was encountering a great deal of pressure and uneasiness.

What's more, because of this, she drank. Even though Anna felt that she was faulty, that there was a significant issue with her, her brain was working precisely how a vast number of long periods of development had molded it to work. She saw feeling restless and afterwards attempted to plan something to cause herself to feel better, which was to drink. This methodology for feeling better improved; however, it just worked incidentally. Since she's an ordinary human, her nervousness returned. And afterwards, what's more, she was currently distraught at herself and blaming herself for her conduct for letting her feeling travelers reroute her transport. What we talked about was that the nervousness wasn't the issue; it was the "arrangement" she used to dispose of it. This is regularly the situation.

We as a whole wind up getting things done to abstain from feeling terrible and a large number of our unhealthy habits feel marvelous for the time being! They are incredibly successful present moment "fixes" for feeling terrible. Are there things you do that assist you with disposing of an inclination in the short run yet meddle with your healthy habits? Possibly it's eating chocolate following an upsetting day. Perhaps it's eating on treats when you're exhausted. Perhaps it's drinking or smoking to unwind. There's nothing broken about what you're doing. People are designed to stay away from torment, and whatever you're doing works in the short run. It's in the drawn-out that these methodologies make issues since they frequently redirect us from our course and like this doesn't assist us with building a healthy life that issues to us.

Simply Don't Worry About It!

Not just has our brain been molded to assist us with staying away from awful sentiments, we get this message in a wide range of routes in Western culture. Friends and family, outsiders, advertisements, the media they all disclose to us that if we simply invested sufficient effort, we'd have the option to change our sentiments, as though we can find ourselves not to feel miserable or stressed or distracted.

We should attempt a psychological test to check whether you can find yourself not to feel restless. Envision that you're in a dunk tank, and the switch that discharges the seat you're perched on is associated with anodes taped to your body. On the off chance that you experience tension, these terminals transfer the data to the switch, activating it to drop you in the pool. To rouse you not to feel restless, the pool is loaded with sharks. All you need to do to abstain from falling into the pool of sharks is not to feel restless. Might you be able to do it? Might anyone be able to do it? Most likely not, despite the great inspiration. But we're continually informed that we ought to have the option to change our emotions. We likewise continually get messages to disregard our emotions or to refute them. My eight-year-old child's school sent him home with a gift depicting a couple of situations for which he expected to think of a curing reaction. The prevailing situation was "Your sister tumbles down and harms herself. She is crying. What would you be able to do?" He stated, "Disclose to her, she's fine." Noooooo! I thought. That is not empathetic by any means! I was shocked!

In any case, soon after that at one of his hockey games, a child tumbled down, and the mentors began hollering, "You're fine! Get up! You're fine!" I understood this was what he'd been instructed to do when somebody was harmed. You don't need to be at a game to watch this kind of conduct. Head over to a play area and trust that a youngster will tumble down. A parent will say, "You're fine." As guardians, we make statements like this to our children always. We don't expect to nullify their emotions, an incredible inverse. We're attempting to cause them to feel better. We're instructing children to overlook, change, or fix their emotions. At the point when it doesn't appear to be alright to feel our sentiments, we regularly take part in unhealthy habits to (briefly) cause the emotions to leave. How about we investigate another alternative. In any case, this identical basic reasoning psyche can, in like manner drive us into trouble. A noteworthy number of us in the mad world don't need to place broad proportions of effort in finding food or water or safe house. Most of the habits in which we deal with these issues are immediate and clear: go to the general store, turn on the tap, turn live broadcasting conditioner. As a result of this relative encourage our necessary reasoning psyche scans for other "issues" to settle, since it's structured. One of various "issues" our brains will Endeavor to fathom is weight, or some other painful condition (for example, diabetes, perpetual torment, coronary sickness). Our primary reasoning cerebrum recognizes weight as an issue and endeavors to get us to settle it or to discard it. Western culture controls our basic deduction cerebrum with messages that weight is intensely affected by us, and if you're overweight, you're a failure, or you're impassive. One of my clients, Claire, was a model instance of someone who experienced negative results as a result of the underlying reasoning cerebrum. Claire depicted to me the different eating regimens, rec focuses, tutors and wellbeing improvement plans she'd used to Endeavor to get fit as a fiddle. Similarly, like others, she had consumed a colossal number of dollars, contributed a gigantic proportion of time and effort, and yielded things she acknowledged to "fix" her weight potentially to end up heavier than when she had started. Sound characteristic?

A key issue with the underlying reasoning cerebrum is that it will all in all focus on the number on the scale as the goal and extent of weight decrease accomplishment. However, using this number alone can indeed provoke some unintended outcomes as time goes on. For example, Claire depicted adding movement to her weight decrease attempts. "Each time I practice I put on weight," she let me know. Since getting fit as a fiddle was her target, her sensible, essential response was to stop rehearsing because it wasn't having any kind of effect. Regardless, we know from ask about that action is noteworthy for extended stretch weight support. Exercise in like manner makes you progressively useful, paying little psyche to your weight. Be that as it may, since training didn't realize sudden weight decrease, Claire showed up at a trademark, evident final product: Why continue rehearsing if it's not helping me show up at my goal? She in this way stopped taking part in that prosperity direct. In any case, whether or not you do get slenderer, focusing on "fixing" your weight regardless of everything has unintended outcomes. Evelyn, another client of mine, adequately shed forty pounds through mindfully counting calories, avoiding every social development including food, and weaving in the evenings (as opposed to eating chips while sitting before the TV). Exactly when she finally got to her goal weight, she was utterly delighted in (Truth, she celebrated by having her favoured food, a solidified yoghurt dessert). Being an overall blended human in Western culture, when she reached her target, she quit managing it and continued forward to the accompanying one. She, as such, quit doing all the practices that helped her get progressively fit.

Notwithstanding the way, this seemed well and well reliant on our perception of targets (taking everything into account, she had accomplished her goal), anyway the practices she was busy with to get slenderer weren't achievable after some time. How was she going to avoid social activities, including food interminably just to manage her weight? Science uncovers to us that procedure with weight-related prosperity rehearses long stretch is essential to supervising weight. Exactly as expected, when Evelyn quit taking an interest in her practices, she started restoring the weight on.

Melanie Johnson

Conclusion

These are the foundation of the Diet of Self-Hypnosis and the reason so many clients have been successful with the programmer. We invited you to literally act like a kid at the start of this book, relearn the delights of your childhood and explore the link between the mind and the body. We said that quick weight loss doesn't impose a diet on you. Instead, it provides the ingredient missing from all other diets. It addresses the role and power of your mind to make any diet or lifestyle change more successful.

you have read many of the ideas and your mind-body has absorbed them into deep memory. It doesn't matter if you can recite all of the ideas or not. They 're there, deep inside your memory, entirely managed by your mind-body, just waiting for activation. Trust your mind and your body.

The subconscious handles it for you, without having to interrupt you with tasks and decisions of thought. Let yourself think again about all the things that it does for you every second about the day. For example, at this very moment your mind-body breathes you, inhales and exhales at the perfect rhythm for your needs. Your mind-body also controls the breathing, digestion, immune responses and a host of other functions of the mind-body.

Your memory role is also controlled by your subconscious, allowing you to forget about it all day long and recall as needed. If you think about yourself while reading a concept, "I wouldn't like that," or "that's not for me," your mind-body puts the idea back on the memory shelf to wait for your permission. The ideas that you talk about, "I 'd love to experience that! "Or" or "I want this! "Your mind-body collects from the shelf of your memory and makes use of it. The more you engage in an activity, the more automatically your mind-body learns to do it for you. Your self-hypnosis brings all of this together for you, making your inspiration, values and goals the formula to follow for your mind-body. Let's look at the critical points regarding self-hypnosis and weight loss. Through recalling the Self-Hypnosis Diet truths, you will become grounded at every stage in your journey to your ideal weight.

Once Realities of Self-Hypnosis and Weight Loss

CPSIA information can be obtained
at www.ICGtesting.com
Printed in the USA
BVHW041809021220
594600BV00023B/225